8/8/91

To Connie Kaplan -

     Our first friend in Manchester —

Best regards.

THE DEVELOPMENT OF MEDICAL

TECHNIQUES AND TREATMENTS

THE
DEVELOPMENT OF MEDICAL
TECHNIQUES AND TREATMENTS

From Leeches to Heart Surgery

Martin Duke, M.D.

INTERNATIONAL UNIVERSITIES PRESS, INC.
Madison ● Connecticut

Library of Congress Cataloging in Publication Data

Duke, Martin.
  The development of medical techniques and treatments: from leeches to heart surgery / Martin Duke.
    p. cm.
  Includes bibliographical references.
  Includes index.
ISBN 0-8236-1232-5
  1. Medicine—History. I. Title.
  [DNLM: 1. Alternative Medicine. 2. Cardiology—trends.
3. Clinical Medicine—trends. WB 100 D877d]
R131.D79 1991
610'.9—dc20
DLC
for Library of Congress   90-4666
                                                              CIP

Manufactured in the United States of America

Contents

SECTION III
ON THE ROAD TO CONTEMPORARY CARDIAC CARE

Acknowledgments

For a physician whose *raison d'être* is the direct care of patients, for whom spare time is rare, and to whom those in need and the telephone always seem to reach out during such moments as are occasionally available, the research for and the writing of this book could only have been accomplished with the invaluable advice and support of many individuals. Appreciation is expressed to Karen Rosenberg, editor of *Practical Cardiology*, for granting permission to use and revise several of the author's contributions to that journal during the years 1983–1988 for inclusion in this book. The staffs of the Yale Medical Historical Library and of the Lyman Maynard Stowe Library at the University of Connecticut Health Center were more than generous with their time in locating reference materials during spur-of-the-moment visits, the timing of which was guided by the unpredictable demands of a medical practice. In response to numerous requests, Diane Neumann, librarian at the Hartford Medical Society, ferreted out the answers to seemingly impossible questions with the well-honed skill and efficiency of the knowledgable professional that she is. Jeannine Cyr Gluck and Anna Salo at the medical library in my own hospital in Manchester were tenacious in tracking down and obtaining copies of articles and reports, many of which were a challenge to locate.

I gratefully acknowledge permission to quote from the following works.

Chapter 1: Baker, A. B. (1971), Artificial respiration, the history of an idea. *Medical History*, 15:336–351 (page 338).
Kounwenhoven, W. B., Jude, J. R., and Knickerbocker, G. G. (1960), Closed-chest cardiac massage. *Journal of the American Medical Association*, 173:1064–1067 (page 1064).
Schechter, D. C. (1971a), Early experience with resuscitation by means of electricity. *Surgery*, 69:360–372 (page 363).

Chapter 4: Richards, Jr., D. W. (1962), Medical priesthoods, past and present. *Transactions of the Association of American Physicians,* 75:1–10 (pages 7–8).

Chapter 7: Galvani, L. (1791), *Commentary on the Effects of Electricity on Muscular Motion,* intr. I. B. Cohen, tr. M. G. Foley [Ames]. Norwalk, CT: Burndy Library, 1953 (pages 45–47).

Chapter 13: Castle, W. B. (1961), The Gordon Wilson Lecture: A century of curiosity about pernicious anemia. *Trans. Amer. Clin. Climatol. Assn.,* 73:54–80 (pages 66–67).

Chapter 14: Dickey, J. (1970), Diabetes. In: *The Eye-beaters, Blood, Victory, Madness, Buckhead and Mercy.* Garden City, NY: Doubleday & Co., Inc. (pages 7–9).

Chapter 15: Cournand, A. (1964), Air and blood. In: *Circulation of the Blood: Men and Ideas,* ed. A. P. Fishman and D. W. Richards. New York: Oxford University Press, pages 3–70 (pages 46, 62).

Chapter 18: Lucia, S. P. (1963), *A History of Wine as Therapy.* Philadelphia and Montreal: J. B. Lippincott Co. (page 105).

Chapter 21: Kreig, M. B. (1964), *Green Medicine: The Search for Plants That Heal.* Chicago, New York, San Francisco: Rand McNally and Co. (pages 319–320).

Chapter 24: Braunwald, E. (1966), Symposium on beta adrenergic receptor blockade: An editorial introduction to the symposium. *American Journal of Cardiology,* 18:303–307 (page 307).

Chapter 27: Levine, S. A., and Harvey, W. P. (1959), *Clinical Auscultation of the Heart.* Philadelphia and London: W. B. Saunders Co. (page 306).
Harken, D. E., Soroff, H. S., Taylor, W. J., Lefemine, A. A., Gupta, S. K., and Lunzer, S. (1960), Partial and complete prostheses in aortic insufficiency. *J. Thorac. Cardiovasc. Surg.,* 40:744–762 (page 748).
Starr, A., and Edwards, M. L. (1961), Mitral replacement: Clinical experience with a ball-valve prosthesis. *Ann. Surg.,* 154:726–740 (page 726).

My daughters Annette, Pamela, and Daniella, living at various times in different cities in the northeastern United States, promptly reacted to "emergency" telephone calls to "quickly" obtain "vital" information from major library resources available to them. Rose Cagianello and Nancy White, my office secretaries, unbelievably found the time to type, decipher, and retype manuscripts while at the same time answering telephone calls, responding to patients, maintaining records, and preparing insurance forms. And finally, none of the preceding could have been done without the support, encouragement, and sense of humor of my wife Juliane in permitting our dining and living rooms to be turned into study and storage facilities for reprints, journals, books, reference files, manuscripts, wastepaper baskets, and other accoutrements needed for preparing a book, and in offering plausible explanations to invited guests and friends as to why a portion of the house was off-bounds and meals and social visits were confined to the kitchen.

To all—thank you.

M.D.

Foreword

> There are, of course, in every calling, those who
> go about the work of the day before them, doing it
> according to the rules of their craft, and asking no
> questions of the past or of the future, or of the aim
> and end to which their special labor is contributing.
> [Oliver Wendell Holmes, 1860, pp. 175–176]

THE writer of history, according to the often quoted mineteenth-century German historian Leopold von Ranke, should tell his story "wie es eigentlich gewesen" (1824, p. 393), as it actually was. This is, of course, one of those counsels of perfection impossible to achieve, for history, the story and interpretation of human events, is remarkably complex and unpatterned, depending usually upon incomplete information; it is the story of another time and other places, of events that, although they touch or present, are gone forever. At best we reconstruct them from the echoes of which Martin Duke writes in his epilogue, just as one reconstructs the action and structure of a heart valve from the echoes that, rather than being heard, are *seen* on the screen in the course of an echocardiographic procedure, hardly a record of things "as they really were"!

Medical history traditionally has been told as a story, beginning in myth, of inexorable progress depending upon the work and genius of great men: history as biography, the lives of the "great doctors." It is also told as the story of human disease, beginning with the diseases that afflicted human beings in paleolithic times, through malaria, plague, small pox, tuberculosis, and cholera, up to the present with its AIDS and Alzheimer's disease, alcoholism and drug addiction, lung cancer and heart disease, osteoporosis and hip fracture. It may be told as the story of scientific discovery, the development of the knowledge of human biology, and the rise of technology. Medical history is part of cultural history, inseparable from the social, economic, and political history of every civilization. It is not limited only to our western tradition; there is a medical history of China and India, of Africa and Polynesia, of the Incas and the Aztecs. There is a history of medicine and disease as seen through the eyes of the sick, and a history illumined by the special insights of the artist and poet, the philosopher and the theologian. It is a story too vast to be told or read all at once.

In this volume Dr. Duke has chosen those familiar techniques and treatments that have made modern medicine possible, using them to provide a point of view for his history, and a point of departure for his readers. While medicine is more than its technology, technology has come to symbolize modern medicine, and some would assert to control it. Indeed, without it, neither modern clinical medicine nor biomedical science could have gone far beyond Hippocrates and Galen, and even they were not without their technologies.

When medical students and practitioners feel curiosity about medicine's past, they are likely to ask questions about its technology rather than about old concepts and definitions of disease such as fueled the ancient debates between the humoralists and solidists. They will wonder how the stethoscope came to be, and how anyone could have thought up the electrocardiograph. Cardiopulmonary resuscitation is an everyday event in a busy teaching hospital, and the technology that makes this drama possible could hardly have fallen together all at once. Compared with the excitement of learning that technology, the ethical and economic issues involved in "do not resuscitate" orders are dreary stuff; that discussion can wait for another day. If the attending physician is very senior, with a birth date somewhere around 1920, he can tell from memory about the electrocardiographic apparatus when it really was a galvanometer with a quartz string whose movements were reflected onto a moving strip of photographic film that had to be developed in a dark room before it could be read. Hardly a bedside monitor! In a few pages Dr. Duke tells the story of the development of this remarkable instrument and introduces the reader to William Einthoven, Sir Thomas Lewis, Frank N. Wilson, James B. Herrick, and others of the "great doctors" of his specialty of cardiology. The student, or practitioner, may learn for the first time the identity of those men signified by the initials in the WPW syndrome.

For a number of reasons, some of which have to do with an increase in awareness of their own mortality, or perhaps with their own place in history, many older physicians begin to cultivate an interest in medical history, some as antiquarians, collecting old books and instruments, others as serious scholars. But most students and practitioners are curious about the past, especially about the origins of the techniques and treatments that they are learning about or use every day. It is this curiosity that these essays will both nurture and satisfy. How often, for example, do we speak of the "atropine-like" effects of some tricyclic compound; how delicious then to drop names like belladonna, deadly nightshade, Jimson weed or mandrake into the conversation, and talk of the antiquity of these "atropine-like" drug plants. Another ramble through the ages that will evoke all sorts of questions and observations are the related stories of leeches and anticoagulants, of hirudin and coumadin, and of the rise and fall of one time acceptable, apparently rational treatments and techniques. What about Broussais and his gastroenteritis and 33,000,000 leeches? What are we confidently doing today that seems so reasonable, but will one day sink so quickly into oblivion?

Hundreds of pages have been written on the uses of medical history, hundreds more on how it should be taught and by whom. What follows in these tales of discovery and research is sure to whet the appetite for more, to answer some of the "how come" questions, which are the beginning of serious inquiry. The medical historian, Lloyd G. Stevenson, noted that, "If curiosity is the parent of 'pure' science, love of the past, or curiosity about it, may be the parent of a kind of history which lacks ulterior motive, which does not set out to be of use to anybody" (1966, p. 17). In some kind of utilitarian sense history cannot always claim to be of use, but surely there can be no ulterior motive in satisfying our curiosity, providing new dimensions to an otherwise flat and quotidian world, in being sometimes inspiring, and always entertaining.

Robert U. Massey, M.D.
Dean Emeritus
University of Connecticut School of Medicine

References

Holmes, O. W. (1860), Currents and counter-currents in medical science. In: *Medical Essays: 1842–1882*. Boston: Houghton Mifflin Company, 1888, pp. 173–208.

Stevenson, L. G. (1966), The "new wave" in the history of medicine. In: *Education in the History of Medicine, Report of a Macy Conference*, ed. J. B. Blake. New York: Hafner Publishing, 1968, pp. 9–18.

Von Ranke, L. (1824), Die Geschichten der romanischen und germanischen Volker. Quoted by F. Gilbert (1987), What Ranke meant. *The American Scholar*, 56:393–397.

Preface

IN reflecting upon education in today's world, Robert Massey wrote: "Not to know what or who came before is like trying to make sense of a novel which we have just opened in the middle" (1987, p. 755). Unfortunately, the never-ending pressures on practitioners and students of the healing arts to continually acquire and refine new vocational and technical skills often limit the time and the opportunities for learning about medical practices of the past. With this in mind, the author has attempted to provide concise and relevant accounts of medical therapies and procedures as they have developed over the years, tailoring them to underscore issues of bygone times that may relate to the present while at the same time avoiding historical minutiae and analysis that so often confounds all but the avid specialist of medical history. It has not been the intent to set forth an exhaustive review of the subjects discussed. Rather, the material selected reflects the tastes, interests, biases, and preferences of the author. It is presented with the intent of being pleasurable to read, informative and balanced in context, and of a length that is appropriate given the time constraints imposed upon many in the medical professions.

With the use of excerpts from the writings of our medical predecessors along with comments from literary sources, readers can identify with and partake of exciting ideas and events as they evolved through the ages. To read the words of Hippocrates on diuretic substances, of Dioscorides on narcotic and hallucinogenic plants, of Thomas Sydenham on treatment with iron and with opium, and of Tissot and of Stokes on therapeutic and preventive exercises; to appreciate and wonder at the imaginative concepts of Brunton and of Souttar during the embryonic years of heart valve surgery, and to take the initial steps with Waller and with Einthoven leading to modern-day electrocardiography; to squirm at the two-thousand-year history of the leech in medical practice, and to be intrigued by the exciting investigations that revealed the benefits of nitroglycerine, anticoagulants, insulin, vitamin B_{12}, and beta blocking agents; to stand in awe at the evolving miracles of heart surgery and of heart transplantation, and to realize the not-so-simple origins of the humble thermometer, of the ubiquitous and vital hypodermic syringe, and of the taken-for-granted instruments for recording blood pressure; and to marvel at the early quixotic attempts at blood transfusion therapy and at electrical stimulation of the heart—to be introduced to the historical background and evolution of past discoveries and events will be to form a profound admiration for the perceptiveness, the imagination, and the remarkable abilities of our medical ancestors. As a result, it becomes possible to understand and apply present-day medical practices with added wisdom and insight.

M.D.

Prologue

Of the numerous medical therapies and technologic advances that have been developed over the centuries, a few are represented in the following pages, selected in part because of their significance in providing the framework from which many current medical practices have evolved, and in part because of the distinctive histories, unusual anecdotal events, and human interest stories with which they have been associated. Perforce, the curiosity, medical background, and personal leanings of the author also played a role in deciding which material to present.

Whenever possible, original sources are quoted at length, not only for historical accuracy but, in addition, to allow the reader to experience the atmosphere of the past from the vantage point of the period in which a particular event was described or discovery was made.

For purposes of organization, each chapter has been placed into one of three general sections, recognizing that this division is at times arbitrary: (1) basic clinical techniques, (2) pharmacologic therapies and other remedies that have been used over an extended period of time, and (3) medical and surgical therapies and diagnostic procedures that relate to contemporary cardiac care.

Section I

The Evolution of Basic Clinical Techniques

THIS section examines the history and evolution of techniques and procedures up to the time they became practical clinical realities. Thus, ventilation, cardiac massage, and electrical defibrillation were developed as individual procedures until the occasion when all three were combined to form the composite that is today recognized as cardiopulmonary resuscitation—CPR. Similarly, the myths and practices associated with blood transfusions through the ages are outlined as this procedure was slowly transformed from a risky and infrequently performed operation to a safe method of treatment used daily again and again. For those in the busy practice of medicine in an era of throw-away syringes, it seems hard to believe that the ubiquitous and much-used hypodermic syringe and needle are of relatively recent origin and were developed only in the mid-nineteenth century.

As a result of Laënnec's excessive modesty and embarrassment and his subsequent invention of the stethoscope, generations of physicians have had available to them a useful diagnostic tool that with training and experience can be applied to maximal advantage. The thermometer, today a standard household item in the United States, was not created in the beginning along with man and other animals, but had to be carefully developed and explained to physicians before the time-honored and less accurate practice of hand thermometry was replaced.

1

Clinically useful instruments for taking and recording the blood pressure introduced a new era in medical diagnostics and therapeutics. The availability of this procedure is no longer limited to a physician's office, and all health-care workers, and often patients themselves, can now determine a blood pressure level almost as readily as they can obtain a temperature. The electrocardiogram, a record of electrical impulses from the heart, evolving as it did in a series of events from Aristotle's observation on electrically charged fish to the accidental movement of a frog's leg to the sophisticated string galvanometer of Einthoven, is an important fixture in medical practice, one without which modern clinical cardiology could not have achieved its high level of success.

It should be with a sense of honest pride as well as modesty and humility that those currently using these techniques and procedures regard themselves as the fortunate heirs and descendants of Laënnec, Blundell, Wunderlich, Korotkov, Einthoven, and others of similar stature.

1

Cardiopulmonary Resuscitation: The Breath of Life

EACH of the three procedures used in cardiopulmonary resuscitation (CPR)—artificial respiration, cardiac massage, and electrical countershock in ventricular fibrillation—has its own history. Interesting and detailed in each instance, the background of these life-saving measures is often little appreciated by those who routinely apply them daily.

Artificial Respiration

Because it is easily observed, the significance of breathing in the maintenance of life was probably recognized in antiquity, as suggested in the *Old Testament*, Genesis 2:7: "then the Lord God formed man of dust from the ground, and breathed into his nostrils the breath of life; and man became a living being." According to Baker (1971, p. 337), Galen, the famous Greek physician of the second century A.D., used bellows to inflate the lungs of a dead animal during the course of an experiment. However, application of this procedure did not appear to have been extended to the living animal.

Little further was added to understanding artificial respiration until the sixteenth century, when the great Flemish anatomist Andreas Vesalius outlined a technique for keeping animals alive after opening the chest cavity. In *De humani corporis fabrica* (Baker, 1971), Vesalius not only described a tracheostomy procedure that made possible the performance of artificial respiration, but also gave a clear picture re-

3

4 *Medical Techniques and Treatments*

lating adequate ventilation to proper heart function, a lesson repeatedly emphasized to all who perform present-day CPR procedures:

> But that life may in a manner of speaking be restored to the animal, an opening must be attempted in the trunk of the trachea, into which a tube of reed or cane should be put; you will then blow into this, so that the lung may rise again and the animal take in air. Indeed, with a slight breath in the case of this living animal the lung will swell to the full extent of the thoracic cavity, and the heart become strong and exhibit a wondrous variety of motions. So, with the lung inflated once and a second time, you examine the motion of the heart by sight and touch as much as you wish. . . .
> With this observed, the lung should again be inflated, and with this device, than which I have learned nothing more pleasing to me in Anatomy, great knowledge of the differences in the beats should be acquired. For when the lung, long flaccid, has collapsed, the beat of heart and arteries appears wavy, creepy, twisting, but when the lung is inflated, it becomes strong again and swift and displays wondrous variations [Baker, 1971, p. 338].

Although numerous physiological experiments were subsequently performed using techniques of artificial ventilation, it was not until the eighteenth century, at a time when drowning became an important public and medical issue, that interest was shown in developing this procedure as a therapeutic measure (Baker, 1971, p. 341). Perhaps one of the most fascinating of the early accounts of artificial ventilation by means of mouth-to-mouth breathing was written by John Fothergill (1712–1780), a London practitioner well-known for his original descriptions of diphtheritic sore throat. Entitled "Observations on a case . . . of recovering a man dead in appearance, by distending the lungs with air," its innovative concepts, published nearly two and a half centuries ago, warrant closer examination. Fothergill began his presentation as follows:[1]

> There are some facts, which, in themselves, are of so great importance to mankind, or which may lead to such useful discoveries, that it would seem to be the duty of every one, under whose notice they fall, to render them as extensively public as it is possible [1745, p. 275].

He then reviewed a case reported by a surgeon, William Tossack, in which a man who was apparently dead after suffocating from smoke inhalation, recovered after receiving mouth-to-mouth resuscitation:

[1]For ease of reading, the author has recast Fothergill's text in modern English rather than the old English of the original.

In these circumstances, the surgeon [Tossack], who relates the affair, applied his mouth close to the patient's, and, by blowing strongly, holding the nostrils at the same time, raised his chest fully by his breath. The surgeon immediately felt six or seven very quick beats of the heart; the thorax continued to play, and the pulse was soon after felt in the arteries. . . . In one hour the patient began to come to himself; within four hours he walked home; and in as many days returned to his work [Fothergill, 1745, p. 276].

Fothergill, a contemporary of the great James Heberden and John Hunter, recognized the uniqueness of this case:

Anatomists, it is true, have long known, that an artificial inflation of the lungs of a dead or dying animal will put the heart in motion, and continue it so for some time; yet this is the first instance I remember to have met with, wherein the experiment was applied to the happy purpose of rescuing life from such imminent danger [Fothergill, 1745, pp. 276–277].

In discussing this experience, Fothergill (1745) mentioned other patients who might respond to this procedure, including those suffocating from "noxious vapours" (p. 278), those "struck dead by lightning, or any violent agitation of the passions, as joy, fear, surprize" (p. 278), and "those who have been suffocated in the water" (p. 279). Responding to a suggestion "that a pair of bellows might possibly be applied with more advantage in these cases, than the blast of a man's mouth," Fothergill commented that "blowing" (p. 280), would seem preferable because:

1st. as the bellows may not be at hand: 2dly, as the lungs of one man may bear, without injury, as great a force as those of another man can exert; which by the bellows cannot always be determin'd: 3dly, the warmth and moisture of the breath would be more likely to promote the circulation, than the chilling air forced out of a pair of bellows [p. 280].

During the nineteenth century and first half of the twentieth century, a variety of manual methods for administering artificial respiration was recommended, particularly for use in victims of drowning (Baker, 1971, pp. 345–346). Controversies raged as to whether patients should be placed in a supine, lateral, or prone position and as to the site on which pressure to the body should be applied. One method required repetitively raising the victim's arms over the head in order to elevate the ribs and enlarge the chest cavity. When the arms were lowered and the chest compressed laterally, expiration was achieved. Another method, the well-known prone-pressure method of artificial respiration, was recommended by Schäfer and was commonly used for many years:

> The operator kneels or squats either across or on one side of the [prone] subject facing the head, and places his hands close together flat upon the back of the subject over the loins, the fingers extending over the lowest ribs. By now leaning forwards upon the hands, keeping the elbows extended, the weight of the operator's body is brought to bear upon the subject, and this not only compresses the lower part of the thorax but also the abdomen against the ground, the pressure being fairly equably distributed. The result of this is that not only is the thorax diminished in extent from before back, but, owing to the pressure which is communicated to the abdomen, the viscera are compressed and tend to force the diaphragm up, so that the thorax is diminished in capacity from above down. . . . The pressure is applied not violently, but gradually, during about three seconds, and is then released by the operator swinging his body back, but without removing his hands. The elasticity of the chest and abdomen cause these to resume their original dimensions and air passes in through the trachea. After two seconds the process is again commenced and is continued in the same way, the operator swinging his body forwards and backwards once every five seconds or about twelve times a minute, without any violent effort and with the least possible exertion [1908, pp. 237–238].

At the same time as such manual methods were in popular use, however, others spoke out in favor of the mouth-to-mouth method of artificial respiration. As far back as 1906, Woods, for one, stated that

> it seems to me to be clear from every consideration that the mouth-to-mouth or nose method gives the patient the best chance, for, to recapitulate:—
> (1) The quantity of tidal air is greater than by any indirect method, and, therefore, the stimulation of the mechanisms of circulation and respiration, the elimination of the poison, and the oxygenation of the blood are all as great as possible.
> (2) The impurities, if present at all, are negligible.
> (3) The method can be applied without a moment's loss of time [1906, p. 141].

The controversy over which technique is best was addressed in a classic experiment by Safar, Escarraga, and Elam (1958). By comparing manual procedures such as the chest-pressure arm-lift and back-pressure arm-lift methods of artificial respiration with mouth-to-mouth and mouth-to-airway insufflation methods, it was established that the latter were more effective and beneficial. Thus, two hundred some years had elapsed since Fothergill had documented the benefits of a "blast of a man's mouth" (1745, p. 280).

Cardiac Massage

In the second half of the nineteenth century, alarmed by the frequency with which cardiac arrest occurred during the administration of chloroform anesthesia, investigators began to search for ways of treating this catastrophic event. Hake, after visiting the laboratory of Professor Moritz Schiff in Florence, mentioned the latter's practice of providing *"artificial circulation"* (1874, p. 242) in animals whose hearts had ceased to beat after chloroform anesthesia: "He [Schiff] lays open the thoracic cavity, and, compressing the passive heart with his fingers, imitates in it the periodic movements of that organ. The circulation is restored, the nerves of the heart recover their force, and the organ finally resumes its spontaneous action" (p. 242). Schiff described the procedure he used:

> [I]f the thorax is opened and at the same time air is insufflated into the lungs, by rhythmical compression of the heart with the hand (care being taken in doing so not to interfere with the coronary circulation) and continuous pressure of the abdominal aorta so as to bring the blood in greater quantity towards the head, it was possible to reestablish the heart beat even up to a period of 11 1/2 minutes after the stoppage of that organ [quoted in Green, 1906, p. 1708].

A few years later, Professor Boehm at the University of Dorpat presented evidence indicating that the circulation of cats could be maintained after cardiac arrest by applying rhythmic pressure to the chest—a form of closed-chest cardiac compression or massage (Boehm, 1878). Thus, within a brief period, experimental research demonstrated the effectiveness of both internal and external methods of cardiac massage. Shortly thereafter, this information was translated into clinical practice, and by the start of the twentieth century, reports were beginning to appear of cases in which these procedures were performed.

Gray (1905) described a technique in which, by way of an incision in the abdomen, the heart was manually massaged through the intact wall of the diaphragm, an approach the author referred to as subdiaphragmatic transperitoneal massage of the heart. The following year, Green (1906) summarized the results in thirty-eight cases culled from the medical literature between 1880 and 1906 as well as two of his own. Various methods of massage were identified: the thoracic approach, in which the chest cavity was opened and the heart massaged or compressed directly, either with or without opening the pericardium;

the transdiaphragmatic approach, in which the abdomen was opened and an incision made in the diaphragm through which the operator's fingers were inserted and cardiac massage or compression performed; the above-mentioned subdiaphragmatic route, in which the operator's hand was inserted into the abdomen and pushed up to the under surface of the diaphragm, defining the heart and compressing it against the posterior thoracic wall, counter pressure being applied with the other hand to the exterior of the chest; and the Crile method, which consisted of pressing rhythmically on the anterior chest wall over the heart, a form of closed-chest cardiac massage. There were nine completely successful results in this series of cases, success being defined as a good or uneventful recovery. The author stated his findings as follows:

> 1. That it has been possible in human beings to restore the heart beat by massage when ordinary measures of resuscitation have failed, even when the massage has not been commenced until the heart had been stopped for 45 minutes, but a definite and complete cure has never yet been effected when this interval has been longer than from seven to eight minutes. 2. In many of the cases the adoption of massage for a period of from 30 seconds to five minutes has been sufficient to restore the heart beat but it has sometimes been necessary to go on with it for 15 minutes or even longer. 3. Artificial respiration and its adjuncts must also continuously be applied, and sometimes it is necessary to persevere with it long after pulsation is restored in order to re-establish the respirations [Green, 1906, p. 1712].

It is well worth reviewing in greater detail the far-reaching work of George Crile from Cleveland, briefly alluded to above. Crile wrote:

> In dogs the forcible rhythmic compression of the thorax over the heart by compressing the heart itself and the great vascular trunks, raises the blood-pressure to a certain extent and thus aids its action. The mere stimulation of the first few compressions has a tendency to make the heart resume automatic action, and a feeble circulation may be maintained by the continuation of the rhythmic pressure upon the chest. . . .
> In adults, and especially in children, something can doubtless be accomplished by forcibly activating the elastic chest wall. With the child flat on its back, pressure should be applied at the rate of about 30 to 40 times a minute [1914, pp. 231–232].

Following a discussion of direct or internal methods available for performing cardiac compression or massage, Crile commented further on the effectiveness of external cardiac compression:

If, instead of a single local pressure, a series of rhythmic pressures upon the thorax and abdomen are made the entire blood stream may be energized and moved, that is to say, the person who makes the rhythmic pressure furnishes an external pseudocardiac action. The author has personally been able to effect a complete circulation in a recently dead subject, producing a radial pulse and bleeding of peripheral vessels, and even to make a blood-pressure of measurable tension (registered by a sphygmomanometer) by the combined effect of a tightly inflated rubber suit covering the lower extremities and the abdomen and strong rhythmic pressure from the broadly extended hands applied upon each side of the chest. Indeed, the face could be made to flush and fade appreciably at will [1914, p. 243].

Crile concluded his discussion with a statement as meaningful today as when it was written three quarters of a century ago:

Whatever the method of resuscitation, the one primary and essential object is to supply the brain with an oxygenated circulation. Artificial respiration can be maintained indefinitely with ease; the heart is rather readily started, but unless cerebral anemia be overcome in less than seven minutes the patient passes into the death that knows no awakening [1914, p. 251].

In spite of the demonstrated effectiveness and advantages of closed-chest (sometimes referred to as indirect or external) cardiac massage or compression, this technique was not widely applied for many years. During the intervening period, open-chest cardiac massage continued to be performed, usually restricted to patients in the hospital and rarely attempted elsewhere. Finally, in 1960, Kouwenhoven, Jude, and Knickerbocker in Baltimore rediscovered and perfected the method of closed-chest massage, demonstrating the effectiveness of appropriately applied pressure over the chest wall in maintaining an adequate flow of blood to vital organs (Figure 1.1). The significance of this work in extending the benefits of cardiac massage and of the resuscitation procedure to a broad rather than to a limited population cannot be overemphasized. The authors wrote:

Cardiac resuscitation after cardiac arrest or ventricular fibrillation has been limited by the need for open thoracotomy and direct cardiac massage. As a result of exhaustive animal experimentation a method of external transthoracic cardiac massage has been developed. Immediate resuscitative measures can now be initiated to give not only mouth-to-nose artificial respiration but also adequate cardiac massage without thoracotomy. The use of this technique on 20 patients has given an over-all permanent survival rate of 70%. Anyone, anywhere, can now initiate cardiac resuscitative procedures. All that is needed are two hands [1960, p. 1064].

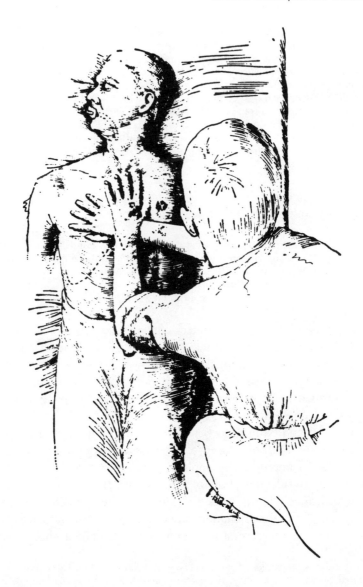

FIG. 1.1. The technique of external or closed-chest cardiac massage, as illustrated by Kouwenhoven, Jude, and Knickerbocker (1960), a procedure that broadened the opportunities for performing cardiac resuscitation. *Source:* Kouwenhoven, W. B., Jude, J. R., and Knickerbocker, G. G. (1960), Closed-chest cardiac massage. *J. Amer. Med. Assn.*, 173:1064–1067, Fig. 2. Copyright 1960, American Medical Association.

Electrical Countershock

The final component of the trilogy of techniques comprising present-day cardiopulmonary resuscitation—electrical countershock for ventricular fibrillation or defibrillation—may have been introduced into clinical practice over two hundred years ago. As described in accounts from the *Registers of the Royal Humane Society of London* for 1774–1784, electroshock therapy applied to the chest was used in resuscitating those apparently dead, although there is no way of knowing whether these patients had cardiac asystole or ventricular fibrillation or some other cardiac arrhythmia. The verbatim report of one such dramatic incident was cited by Schechter:

> One part of our benevolent design is to manifest the possibility of recovery in the various instances of sudden death, where the vital powers are suspended, without any essential injury to the frame. This extraordinary relation of resuscitation also manifests the admirable powers of the electrical shock; which we would earnestly recommend in all cases of suspended animation.
> Sophia Greenhill, on Thursday last, fell out of a one-pair-of-stairs window, and was taken up by a man to all appearance dead. The surgeons at the Middlesex Hospital, and an apothecary, declared that nothing could be done for the child.—Mr. Squires, tried the effects of electricity.—Twenty minutes elapsed before he could apply the shock, which he gave to various parts of the body in vain;—but, upon transmitting a few shocks through the thorax, he perceived a small pulsation; in a few minutes the child began to breathe with great difficulty, and after some time she vomited.—A kind of stupor, occasioned by the depression of the cranium, remained for several days, but, by the proper means being used, her health was restored [1971a, p. 363].[2]

Allan Burns of Glasgow (1781–1813), one of the first physicians to appreciate the relationship of angina pectoris to myocardial ischemia, suggested the clinical application of electric shock therapy in patients with heart disease and cardiac arrest:

> Where however, the cessation of vital action is very complete, and continues long, we ought to inflate the lungs, and pass electric shocks through the chest: the practitioner ought never, if the death has been sudden, and the person not very far advanced in life, to despair of success, till he has unequivocal signs of real death [1809, pp. 147–148].

John Alexander McWilliam (1857–1937), Professor of Physiology

[2]Reproduced from *Surgery*, Vol. 69, pp. 360–372 (specifically p. 363), by D. C. Schechter, 1971.

at the University of Aberdeen in Scotland, in discussing the causes of ventricular fibrillation—a condition known at the time by such names as "Herz-delirium, Delirium cordis, Fibrillar contraction, Intervermiform movement" (McWilliam, 1887, p. 296)—wrote:

> The state of arhythmic fibrillar contraction is essentially due to certain changes occurring within the ventricles themselves. It is not due to the passage of any abnormal nerve impulses to the ventricles from other parts, or to the interruption of any impulses normally transmitted to the ventricles and necessary for their normal co-ordinated action. The condition is not due to injury or irritation of the nerves that pass over the ventricles from the base of the heart [p. 297].

McWilliam added later in his discussion:

> The state of arhythmic fibrillar contraction . . . appears to be constituted by a rapid succession of inco-ordinated [sic] peristaltic contractions—a condition that can be brought about either (1) by the influence of certain depressing or paralysing agents upon the ventricular tissue, or (2) by the application of certain forms of stimulation to the ventricular tissue [p. 308].

In experiments performed at the turn of the twentieth century, Prévost and Battelli from Geneva demonstrated that an electrical discharge applied directly to the heart of an animal in ventricular fibrillation can restore the rhythm to normal (Stephenson, 1974, pp. 240–241). These studies, unfortunately, were little noted for over twenty-five years until, as later recounted by William Kouwenhoven and Orthello Langworthy (1973), a series of events established their medical significance. Concerned by the increasing number of deaths and accidents occurring in linemen and among the public as a result of electric shocks and the ensuing problems of cardiac and respiratory arrest, Dr. Lieb of the Consolidated Edison Company of New York approached the Rockefeller Institute in 1926 for advice on how to reduce this high fatality rate. Several committees were assigned to study the problem, including a group led by Professor William H. Howell of the Johns Hopkins University. Howell asked a question of the multidisciplinary team working with him—Hooker, Langworthy, and Kouwenhoven, a physiologist, a neurologist, and an electrical engineer respectively—about the long-neglected work of Prévost and Battelli, "Is it true?" (Kouwenhoven and Langworthy, 1973, p. 187). The extensive investigations that followed answered this question in the affirmative: "With the electrodes applied directly to the heart [of a dog], currents of 0.4 ampere for five seconds will cause fibrillation and currents of 0.8 ampere or more will stop fibrillation" (Hooker, Kouwenhoven, and Langworthy, 1933, p. 454).

Further research over the years by these investigators and their associates at Johns Hopkins, together with fundamental studies by Carl Wiggers and René Wégria in Cleveland (1940) on the increased susceptibility of the heart to ventricular fibrillation during the vulnerable period of the cardiac cycle, paved the way for the first successful report of electrical defibrillation in a human, a fourteen-year-old boy in whom ventricular fibrillation developed at the time of chest surgery and who, following the application of electric shocks directly to the heart, recovered completely (Beck, Pritchard, and Feil, 1947).

During the late 1930s, Gurvich and Yuniev in the Soviet Union developed a technique whereby "Momentary electrical stimulation of the fibrillating heart by a condenser discharge abolishes [ventricular] fibrillation" (1946, p. 238), the electrical shock being applied through the intact chest wall of the animal without surgically exposing the heart. The same investigators also made the following significant comments about the duration of cardiac arrest, the use of cardiac massage, and the ability to defibrillate the heart:

> The condenser discharge restored cardiac function if the discharge was applied not later than 1–1 1/2 minutes after the onset of fibrillation. However, this interval of time does not constitute the limit. By means of preliminary massage of the heart, normal cardiac function may be restored by discharges applied after a rather long period of fibrillation [Gurvich and Yuniev, 1947, pp. 254–255].

Thus, effective cardiac massage was shown to prolong the period of time during which successful defibrillation might still take place. Unfortunately, much of the work of these Russian investigators, although reported in the foreign medical literature during the late 1930s, was not available in the previously quoted English medical publications until after World War II.

By the mid-1950s, a group of investigators at Harvard Medical School (Zoll, Linenthal, Gibson, Paul, and Norman, 1956) and a team at the Johns Hopkins University (Kouwenhoven, Milnor, Knickerbocker, and Chesnut, 1957) independently developed clinically useful instruments for closed-chest defibrillation and applied them successfully in several patients. The importance of these devices was evident to all and their adoption by the medical profession was immediate.

In the 1960s, with the effectiveness of mobile-intensive care units having been demonstrated by Pantridge and Geddes in Belfast, Ireland (1967), the benefits of CPR spread from the hospital to the community at large. At this point, most of the basic work on cardiac arrest and resuscitation had been done, and what remained was principally a matter of refining technology and of extending the educational opportunities to a larger group of people so that, as cited above "Anyone, anywhere, can now initiate cardiac resuscitative procedures. All that is needed are two hands" (Kouwenhoven, Jude, and Knickerbocker, 1960, p. 1064).

The marvel of cardiopulmonary resuscitation was recognized and acknowledged by many, including William Kouwenhoven, a pioneer in this field, who wrote in a publication that discussed his own vital role in the development of the defibrillator:

> The discovery and development of cardiopulmonary resuscitation made the closed-chest defibrillator a useful and effective device for depolarizing fibrillating human hearts. Many lives have been saved, and I thank the Lord for the opportunity that has been granted me [1969, p. 457].

The awesome responsibility of being able to partake in the miracle of bringing about "the breath of life" (Genesis 2:7) had been granted to man.

2

The Early Years of Blood Transfusions

For the life of the flesh is in the blood.
[Leviticus, 17:11]

FROM biblical and ancient Roman times to the present, blood has been regarded as synonymous with life. In the belief that blood contained the physical and mental qualities of the person in whom it flowed, it was common practice in ancient Rome to drink the blood of fallen gladiators in order to acquire their strength. A similar attempt to rejuvenate an aged Pope Innocent VIII by giving him the blood of three young boys was recorded in 1492 (Hutchin, 1968, p. 685). Over the years, the value of blood as food has been recognized, with Marco Polo having observed Mongol soldiers "living only on the blood of their horses" (Tannahill, 1973, p. 130) on long marches, a practice not unlike that of present-day African Masai tribesmen of drinking the blood of their cattle. Similarly, during the late nineteenth century in France, ladies went to slaughterhouses to ingest blood for medicinal purposes (Tannahill, 1973, p. 342). Thus, throughout history, many societies have attributed a health and nutritional value to the administration of human and animal blood.

In the mid-seventeenth century, Sir Christopher Wren, architect of London's famous churches, injected opium, wine, and beer into the veins of dogs by means of a primitive syringe made of a quill and a dog's bladder (Hutchin, 1968, p. 686). A few years later, in 1664, a physician and professor of anatomy and botany at the University of Kiel named Johannes Daniel Major described the effects produced in animals by the intravenous injection of medications. According to Brown, however, Major felt "that his experiments had proved to be of but little value, and that the danger of their action was greater than any benefit derived from them" (1917, p. 183).

It was these early studies that suggested to others the possibility of transfusing blood into the veins of animals. During the seventeenth century, a report of such a procedure was incorporated by Richard Lower of Oxford in his famous *Tractatus de Corde* which was translated from the original Latin by K. J. Franklin:

> For many years at Oxford I saw others at work, and myself, for the sake of experiment, injected into the veins of living animals various opiate and emetic solutions, and many medicinal fluids of that sort. The technical procedure for this is now quite well known, and this is not the place to describe the individual results and outcomes of these experiments. But when, in addition, I likewise injected many nutrient solutions, and had seen the blood of different animals mix quite well and harmoniously with various injections of wine and beer, it soon occurred to me to try if the blood of different animals would not be much more suitable and would mix without danger or conflict. And, because in shed blood (no matter how well coagulation should be guarded against by repeated shaking) the natural blending and texture of the parts must of necessity change, I thought it much more convenient to transfer the unimpaired blood of an animal, which was still alive and breathing, into another [Lower, 1669, pp. 172–173].

Lower described his now-famous transfusion experiment as follows:

> Having got ready the dogs, and made other preparations as required, I selected one dog of medium size, opened its jugular vein, and drew off blood, until it was quite clear from its howls and struggles that its strength was nearly gone and that convulsions were not far off. Then, to make up for the great loss of this dog by the blood of a second, I introduced blood from the cervical artery of a fairly large mastiff, which had been fastened alongside the first dog, until this latter animal by its restiveness showed in its turn that it was overfilled and burdened by the amount of the inflowing blood. I ligatured the artery from which the blood was passing, and withdrew blood again from the receiving dog. This was repeated several times in succession, until there was no more blood or life left in two fairly large mastiffs (the blood of both having been taken by the smaller dog). In the meantime blood had been repeatedly withdrawn from this smaller animal and injected into it in such amount as would equal, I imagine, the weight of its whole body, yet, once its jugular vein was sewn up and its binding shackles cast off, it promptly jumped down from the

table, and, apparently oblivious of its hurts, soon began to fondle its master, and to roll on the grass to clean itself of blood; exactly as it would have done if it had merely been thrown into a stream, and with no more sign of discomfort or of displeasure [1669, pp. 174–176].

With the aid of illustrations, Lower explained the technique and the equipment used to connect the artery of a donor dog with the vein of a recipient animal (1669, pp. 185–188). He followed this account with a unique discussion of a transfusion from a sheep to a man, performed in order to change the patient's mental condition.

> For there is no reason to think that the blood of other animals mixes less well with human blood than with animal blood. This view is abundantly confirmed by recent experiments of French workers; and I also found it so not very long ago in the case of a certain A.C., who was the subject of a harmless form of insanity. I superintended the introduction into his arm at various times of some ounces of sheep's blood at a meeting of the *Royal Society*, and that without any inconvenience to him. In order to make further experiments on him with some profit also to himself, I had decided to repeat the treatment several times in an effort to improve his mental condition [1669, pp. 189–190].

The uniqueness and creativity of such experiments (Figure 2.1) were not lost on Samuel Pepys, an English government official but far better remembered as an accurate chronicler of London life during the second half of the seventeenth century. On November 14, 1666, Pepys made the following entry in his now-famous diary:

> Dr. Croone told me, that, at the meeting at Gresham College to-night, which, it seems, they now have every Wednesday again, there was a pretty experiment of the blood of one dog let out, till he died, into the body of another on one side, while all his own run out on the other side. The first died upon the place, and the other very well, and likely to do well. This did give occasion to many pretty wishes, as of the blood of a Quaker to be let into an Archbishop, and such like; but, as Dr. Croone says, may, if it takes, be of mighty use to man's health, for the amending of bad blood by borrowing from a better body [1666–1668, pp. 10–11].

While this work was under way in England, several sheep-to-man blood transfusions were being performed in France by Jean-Baptiste Denis (also referred to as Denys or Dionys). However, with the death of one of these patients, Denis was brought to trial for manslaughter. Although he was acquitted of the charge, it was decided to prohibit further blood transfusions in France, a decision also made in several other European countries (Maluf, 1954; Hutchin, 1968). The stage

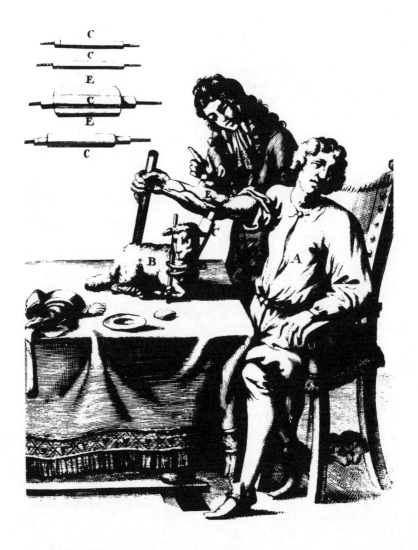

FIG. 2.1. An idealized illustration of a transfusion from a lamb to a man, from a German surgical textbook of the late seventeenth century. *Source:* Purmann, M. G. (1692), *Grosser und gantz neugewundener Lorbeer-Krantz.* Courtesy of the National Library of Medicine, History of Medicine Division, Bethesda, MD.

was not yet set for the rational and scientific use of transfusions. As Maluf stated: "It is probably fortunate that blood transfusion took a nap for over one and a half centuries. Ignorance of antisepsis, asepsis, and immunology would have resulted in countless disasters had blood not clotted readily and had transfusions been frequent" (1954, p. 67).

Until the first half of the nineteenth century, little if any serious consideration appeared to have been given to administering a transfusion to a patient in whom loss of blood had occurred. Somewhat surprisingly, it was an obstetrician and lecturer at St. Thomas's Hospital and Guy's Hospital in London named James Blundell who was inspired to institute a series of well planned and original studies that eventually led to the use of human blood transfusions for patients with severe hemorrhage. Blundell's ability to perform these difficult experiments and the remarkably accurate conclusions that he was able to draw from them, particularly in the absence of any pertinent knowledge of blood coagulation and immunology, can best be appreciated by referring to his own words:

> A few months ago I was requested to visit a woman who was sinking under uterine hemorrhagy [sic]. The discharge had stopped before my arrival, but her fate was decided, and notwithstanding every exertion of the medical attendants, she died in the course of two hours.
> Reflecting afterwards on this melancholy scene, for there were circumstances which gave it a peculiar interest, I could not forbear considering, that the patient might very probably have been saved by transfusion [1818, p. 56].

Rather than going immediately to the bedside of patients to study this problem, Blundell (1818) performed his initial experiments in the animal laboratory. There he was able to demonstrate that blood does not lose its properties after passing through a syringe or other instrumentation, that venous blood is as satisfactory as arterial blood for transfusion purposes, and "that it is not necessary in cases of haemorrhagy to throw into the vessels as much blood as they have lost; a very small supply, although it will not restore the energies of the animal, will preserve its life" (1818, p. 75). Perhaps Blundell's most significant contribution was made when, after noting the death of animals that had received transfusions of human blood, he warned of the dangers of transfusing blood between different species (heterologous blood transfusion):

> But of all the advantages derived from transfusion by the syringe, by far the

most important is the opportunity it offers of throwing human blood into human veins. There seems reason for surmising, from facts already related, that the blood of one class of animals cannot be substituted, in large quantities, for that of another with impunity; and hence it becomes of the utmost importance, that we should be able to supply the human vessels with the human blood. Every other method of transfusion with which I am acquainted, is exposed to this grand objection, that it transfuses the blood of the brute—a defect, from which the operation by the syringe is *exclusively* exempt [1818, p. 75].

Rather than using the difficult and cumbersome procedure of transfusing blood by connecting a donor directly to a recipient, Blundell designed instruments for first collecting blood and then administering it by the so-called method of indirect transfusion (Figure 2.2). Most importantly, he was able to show that no damage occurred to the blood as it passed through these instruments, either a form of syringe (Blundell, 1818) or an apparatus called a "Gravitator" (Blundell, 1828–1829b). The following excerpt from a description of a patient with severe post-partum hemorrhage captures the uniqueness and formidable nature of the transfusion procedure as it was then performed (perhaps rightfully referred to as an operation) and the awe with which it was regarded by both physician and patient:

An alarming state of collapse somewhat suddenly ensued, and it was found that considerable haemorrhage had taken place from the uterus. . . . [H]e [Dr. Blundell] thought the balance was against her, and that it was desirable to give the pabulum vitae,—*blood*. About eight ounces, procured from the arm of Mr. Davies, were injected at different times—the whole operation occupying upward of three hours. . . . It is worthy of notice, that the patient expresses herself very strongly on the benefits resulting from the injection of the blood; her observations are equivalent to this—that she felt as if *life* were infused into her body [1828–1829a, pp. 431–432].

Before blood transfusions could be considered safe and clinically useful, immunological problems still needed to be defined, and a suitable way to prevent blood from clotting had to be found.

Independent observations by two German investigators in the 1870s, Emil Ponfick and Leonard Landois, described the hazards of transfusions between different species, noting destruction of red blood cells, the resultant appearance of hemoglobin in the urine, and the occurrence of kidney damage and shutdown (Maluf, 1954, pp. 81–85). Their observations provided an explanation for Blundell's findings of more than fifty years before regarding the dangers of such transfusions,

Tab. 1.

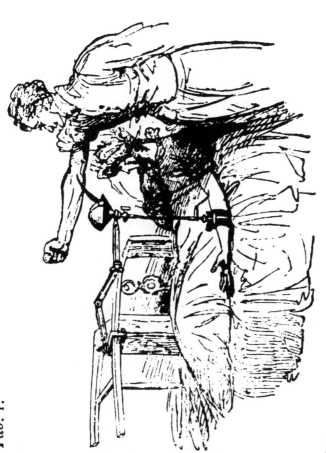

No. 302.

FIG. 2.2. The first transfusion of human blood to a patient has been attributed to James Blundell. In this sketch from one of his early nineteenth-century publications, blood from the vein of a standing donor flows into an instrument; it was called a "Gravitator" because gravity provided the force to propel the blood from it into the vein of the supine patient. *Source:* Blundell, J. (1828–1929), Observations on transfusion of blood by Dr. Blundell with a description of his Gravitator. *Lancet,* 2:321–324.

and effectively ended any further use of blood transfusions in clinical practice between animals and humans.

At the start of the twentieth century, it was recognized that homologous blood transfusions, that is, transfusions between individuals of the same species, may at times also result in the destruction of red blood cells. Samuel Shattock in England observed that human red blood cells could be agglutinated (clumped) by the sera of another individual (Shattock, 1900). However, he attributed this phenomenon to the diseases present in the patients being examined. The following year, Karl Landsteiner, then an assistant in the Institute of Pathological Anatomy at the University of Vienna, reported that serum of given individuals agglutinated the red blood cells obtained from certain other persons (1901). His work in recognizing the presence of three blood groups—the fourth and rarest group was described the following year by Decastello and Sturli (1902)—prepared the way for safer blood transfusions in later years. A superb discussion of this subject can be found in Landsteiner's Nobel Lecture entitled "Individual Differences in Human Blood," read in Stockholm in 1930 on the occasion of his receiving the Prize for Medicine for contributions to this field (Landsteiner, 1931).

During the early years of the twentieth century, Reuben Ottenberg at the Mount Sinai Hospital in New York City applied Landsteiner's work to clinical medicine. His efforts were instrumental in educating physicians as to the importance of cross-matching blood before giving a transfusion:

> It is possible, by methods now known, to determine beforehand whether hemolysis is likely to occur when any two given bloods are mixed. . . . A test of this kind, and a better knowledge of the diseases which contraindicate transfusion, should make transfusion one of the safest and most valuable of therapeutic measures [Ottenberg, 1908, p. 505].

A few years later, these findings were reemphasized: "Accidents in transfusion due to the occurrence of hemolysis or agglutination of the donor's blood-cells by the patient's serum, or vice versa, can be absolutely excluded by careful preliminary blood-tests. We have been able to prevent accidents of this kind in 125 transfusions" (Ottenberg and Kaliski, 1913, p. 2140). Several more years were to elapse, however, before cross-matching blood prior to transfusion became a universally accepted standard of care.

Ever since the first transfusions were attempted, clotting during the procedure had been a major problem. In 1821, two Frenchman, Jean Louis Prévost and Jean Baptiste André Dumas, demonstrated that blood coagulation could be prevented by defibrination, an awkward approach in which blood was stirred or whipped to remove fibrin. In the absence of any other technique, however, this practice remained in use until the turn of the century (Hutchin, 1968, p. 692). John Braxton Hicks, another well-known obstetrician who followed in the footsteps of Blundell at Guy's Hospital, attempted to transfuse blood that had been made incoagulable when mixed with a chemical —phosphate of soda (1869). Unfortunately, all the patients receiving blood prepared in this way died soon after the transfusion, although "[I]n all these cases, as far as the performance of the operation [the transfusion procedure] itself was concerned, the difficulties [due to clotting] were remarkably reduced" (Hicks, 1869, p. 13). Whether the added chemical had a toxic effect and may have contributed to the fatal outcome of these patients is not clear. This, however, was one of the earliest attempts at adding a chemical agent to donors' blood in order to prevent clotting and facilitate the transfusion procedure.

It has been known since the last decade of the nineteenth century that calcium was essential in order for blood coagulation to occur, and that clotting did not take place if certain chemicals that bound with calcium were added to blood (Arthus and Pagès, 1890). Almost twenty-five years later, citrated blood was introduced into clinical medicine by Hustin of Belgium (1914) and Lewisohn in the United States (1916), among others. Lewisohn demonstrated the appropriate amount of the chemical that would not cause toxicity when administered to a human being but would at the same time be adequate as an anticoagulant in the transfused blood:

> The 0.2 per cent. dose, therefore, allows us to transfuse as much as 2500 c.c. of blood at a time, and that is more than anybody ever wants to take from a donor or introduce into the recipient. My experiences with citrate transfusion in children are the best proof of the atoxicity of the citrate method and the 0.2 per cent. dose [1916, p. 619].

By adding glucose to blood, Rous and Turner (1916) demonstrated that the life-span of red blood cells could be prolonged, thus permitting blood withdrawn from a donor to be kept for a longer period of time before being transfused. Oswald Robertson used solutions of citrate and glucose to preserve adequate quantities of blood at the battlefront during World War I, describing what might be called the first blood bank:

> As first found by Rous and Turner, it is possible to preserve living human red blood cells for several weeks in a solution of dextrose and citrate, when kept at ice-box temperature. This method of keeping blood has been made use of recently for giving transfusions at casualty clearing stations during a rush period. A quantity of blood was stored up beforehand ready for use when needed. The blood was kept for varying periods up to twenty-six days before transfusion. Twenty-two transfusions were given to twenty cases by this method. The majority of these were cases of haemorrhage. The results of preserved blood transfusion were quite as striking as those seen after transfusion with blood freshly drawn. There was the same marked improvement, the patients stood operation well, and subsequent progress was quite as good as in those cases transfused by the usual methods. The introduction of kept red blood cells had no apparent harmful effect, as there were no reactions or evidence of increased haemolysis after transfusion.
>
> The chief advantage of this method over other methods of transfusion in current use is the great convenience of having a stock of blood on hand for busy times. The transfusions can be given relatively quickly, and the technique, which is simple and easily acquired, can be carried out entirely by one medical officer.
>
> Experiments in the transportation of preserved blood have shown that it can be carried a considerable distance without injury [Robertson, 1918, p. 695].

During the period between World Wars I and II, Yudin in Russia demonstrated that cadaver blood could be stored and later transfused (1936). This idea met with considerable resistance in many parts of the world, although the increasing recourse to organ transplantation in recent years may yet make this an economically, technically, socially, and legally acceptable procedure (Swan and Schechter, 1962).

The observations that blood could be stored safely for prolonged periods of time led to an expanding interest in blood banks. Bernard Fantus, director of therapeutics at Cook County Hospital in Chicago, is credited with founding the first such facility in the United States (1937). Since World War II, additional improvements in blood transfusion techniques have taken place to meet the demands and high standards of today's complex surgical and medical care. The necessary attention given to the screening of blood donors and the use of various components of blood rather than whole blood have added further dimensions to transfusion therapy.

3

Syringes and Hypodermic Injections

THE skin has long been used by physicians as a pathway for administering medication, with prescriptions written 4,000 years ago
for salves and filtrates having been discovered on a clay tablet in
excavations in the Near East (Kramer, 1954).

Howard-Jones (1947) and Haller (1981) described the origins of
hypodermic medications during the early years of the nineteenth century. A form of therapy identified as iatraliptic treatment consisted of
vigorously rubbing a substance onto the skin surface in the hope that
it would enter the body. In an attempt to further improve absorption,
Lesieur and Lembert introduced the endermic method of therapy—the
application of blisters and caustics to remove the epidermis or super-
ficial layers of the skin, following which the medication in the form
of a powder, solution, or medicated dressing was placed on the raw
surface. A few years later, in 1836, Lafargue went one step further by
moistening the tip of a vaccination-lancet with morphine, forcing the
instrument horizontally beneath the skin, and keeping it there for a
few seconds while the medication was absorbed, a practice similar to
that used in vaccinating for cowpox. However, these procedures at
times were difficult to perform and were often uncomfortable, with
results that were not always predictable.

It is not clear to whom the honors should be given for initially
developing a syringe for the purpose of administering medications
beneath the skin (a subcutaneous or hypodermic injection). Perhaps
credit should be distributed among several individuals, each of whom
made a worthwhile and somewhat different contribution. Howard-
Jones (1947, p. 237) mentioned two New York physicians, Taylor and

Washington, who claimed that in 1839 they made an incision into the skin through which morphine was injected into subcutaneous tissue with an Anel's syringe, a small instrument with a tapered nozzle initially designed for insertion into a tear duct (Schwidetzky, 1944, p. 34). However, precedence for first using and describing the hypodermic insertion of medication has usually been given to the surgeon Francis Rynd, a colleague of the well-known trio of Irish physicians Corrigan, Stokes, and Graves. Writing about a patient with neuralgia, Rynd stated:

> On the 3rd of June a solution of fifteen grains of acetate of morphia, dissolved in one drachm of creosote, was introduced to the supra-orbital nerve, and along the course of the temporal, malar, and buccal nerves, by four punctures of an instrument made for the purpose. In the space of a minute all pain (except that caused by the operation, which was very slight,) had ceased [1845, pp. 167–168].

It was not until sixteen years later that Rynd described and illustrated this rudimentary syringe in greater detail (Figure 3.1):

> The cannula (A) screws on the instrument at (B); and when the button (C), which is connected to the needle (F), and acted on by a spring, is pushed up (as in Fig 2), the small catch (D) retains it in its place. The point of the needle then projects a little beyond the canula (Fig 2). The fluid to be applied is now to be introduced into the canula through the hole (E), either from a common writing-pen or the spoon-shaped extremity of a silver director; a small puncture through the skin is to be made with a lancet, or the point of the instrument itself is to be pressed through the skin, and on to the depth required; light pressure now made on the handle raises the catch (D), the needle is released, and springs backwards, leaving the canula empty, and allowing the fluid to descend. If the instrument be slowly withdrawn, the parts it passes through, as well as the point to which it has been directed, receive the contained fluid; and still more may be introduced, if deemed expedient [1861, p. 13].

These descriptions by Rynd were unfortunately contained within short reports that were little noticed, and it was not until the carefully documented work of Alexander Wood of Edinburgh that the syringe became better known. Like Rynd, Wood had also conceived of using a subcutaneously administered injection of morphine for the relief of neuralgia. Perhaps the story is best continued in his own words:

> Having occasion, however, about the end of 1853, to endeavour to remove a naevus [a skin lesion] by injection with the acid solution of perchloride of iron, I procured one of the elegant little syringes, constructed for this purpose by

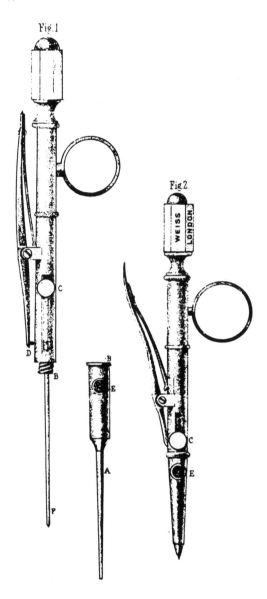

FIG. 3.1. The first hypodermic syringe, used by Francis Rynd of Ireland in 1845, as illustrated and described by him at a later date (1861). *Source:* Rynd, F. (1861), Description of an instrument for the subcutaneous introduction of fluids in affections of the nerves. *Dublin Quarterly J. Med. Sci.*, 32:13. Plate 3.

Mr. Ferguson of Giltspur Street, London. While using this instrument for the naevus, it occurred to me that it might supply the means of bringing some narcotic to bear more directly than I had hitherto been able to accomplish on the affected nerve in neuralgia. I resolved to make the attempt. . . .

I inserted the syringe within the angle formed by the clavicle and acromion, and injected twenty drops of a solution of muriate of morphia. . . . [F]rom that time to this the neuralgia has not returned [1855, pp. 266–267].

On the basis of this and several other cases, Wood concluded:

1st, That narcotics injected into the neighbourhead [*sic*] of the painful point of a nerve affected with neuralgia, will diminish the sensibility of that nerve, and in proportion diminish or remove pain.

2d, That the effec*t* [*sic*] of narcotics so applied are not confined to their local action, but that they reach the brain through the venous circulation, and there produce their remote effects.

3d, That in all probability what is true in regard to narcotics would be found to be equally true in regard to other classes of remedies.

4th, That the small syringe affords a safe, easy, and almost painless method of exhibition [1855, pp. 280–281].

Wood later modified the Ferguson syringe, describing his own instrument as follows:

It [the instrument] consists of a small glass syringe graduated like a drop measure, and to this is attached a small needle, hollow, and having an aperture near the point like the sting of a wasp. The painful point being ascertained, the syringe, being charged, is pressed firmly in to such a depth as to reach the nerve, when the piston being shoved home, the charge is delivered [1858, p. 723].

Thus the basic components of the syringe as it is known today, particularly the hollow needle, became available.

Charles Hunter, house-surgeon at St. George's Hospital, noted that repetitive injections into the same area using Wood's method led to abscess formation. Based upon these observations, additional studies were done resulting in the following report:

Hence he [Hunter] was led to make experiments with a view of discovering whether the action of the remedy depended on its localisation at the painful spot, or whether it would also give relief if injected into other parts of the cellular tissue. The latter turned out to be the case, so that Dr. Wood's remedy proved even more widely applicable than its author had at first supposed [Hunter, 1859, p. 19].

Thus, it was now demonstrated that direct injections into a painful area were unnecessary in order to be effective, and relief of pain could

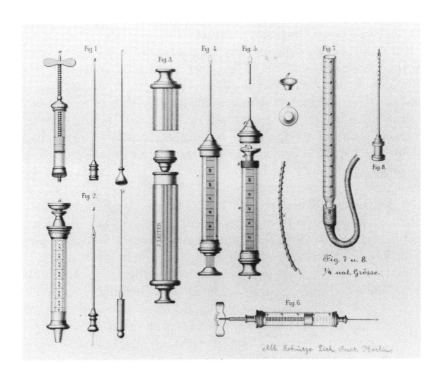

FIG. 3.2. Illustrations of a variety of hypodermic syringes, as depicted in a German textbook from the last half of the nineteenth century, including syringes of Pravaz ("Fig. 1" in the illustration), Luer ("Fig. 2"), and Mathieu ("Fig. 6"). *Source*: Eulenburg, A. (1875), *Die Hypodermatische Injection der Arzneimittel*. Berlin: von August Hirschwald. Courtesy of Yale Medical Historical Library, New Haven, CT.

be obtained as readily by injecting medications at a location distant from the area of discomfort. Hunter also apparently introduced the term "hypodermic" to indicate treatment carried on under the skin (Howard-Jones, 1947, p. 222).

The story of the syringe would be incomplete without mentioning the contributions made by Charles Pravaz and others in France during the last half of the nineteenth century (Howard-Jones, 1947). While involved in the experimental treatment of aneurysms, Pravaz had a syringe made for purposes of injecting a chemical coagulant, iron perchloride, directly into an aneurysm sac in order to form a firm clot and obliterate the lumen. This instrument, consisting of an exploring trocar (sharp-pointed instrument) and cannula or hollow tube to which a small platinum syringe could be attached, was later modified by Béhier for hypodermic use. In later years, famous French instrument makers such as Charrière, Mathieu, and Luer, added further changes in design (Figure 3.2) (Howard-Jones, 1947).

Dr. Fordyce Barker of New York obtained a Ferguson syringe in 1856 while on a trip to Scotland. Using this model, the first hypodermic syringes made in the United States were produced by George Tiemann and Company of New York (Schwidetzky, 1944). The famous Luer all-glass syringe was invented and made about 1896 by Karl Schneider, instrument maker for H. Wulfing Luer of Paris. The right to make this instrument in the United States was acquired shortly thereafter by Becton, Dickinson and Company (Schwidetzky, 1944). Additional design modifications followed, ultimately leading to the present-day industry of disposable syringes.

The hypodermic syringe also fostered the development of many new medications and biological products that are inactivated when administered by mouth and are effective only when given by injection directly into the body. The almost immediate benefits of medications introduced into subcutaneous tissues or directly into the vascular system are among the "miracles" of modern medicine. Thus, it is readily evident how indebted the present-day practice of medicine and surgery is to these omnipresent syringes and needles. The use of these same syringes and needles by narcotic addicts and the contribution of these instruments to the spread of disease such as hepatitis and AIDS are unfortunate by-products with which society is having to cope and for which answers are being sought.

4

Listening to the Sounds of the Body: The Development of the Stethoscope

With the stethoscope René Laënnec first heard the
language of pathology.
[Willius and Keys, 1941, p. 326]

PRIOR to the development of the stethoscope in the early nineteenth
century, physicians had limited means with which to diagnose
chest disorders. According to Garrison (1929, p. 98), the method of
direct auscultation—the application of the ear directly upon the chest
to hear the sounds within—was known to Hippocrates (460–370 B.C.)
in ancient Greece. The value of auscultation was realized by Robert
Hooke (1635–1703) when he wrote:

> Who knows, I say, but that it may be possible to discover the Motions of the
> Internal Parts of Bodies, whether Animal, Vegetable or Mineral, by the sound
> they make, that one may discover the Works perform'd in the severals Offices
> and Shops of a Man's Body, and thereby discover what Instrument or Engine
> is out of order. . . . I have been able to hear very plainly the beating of a Man's
> Heart [1705, p. 39].

In most cases, however, sounds heard by direct auscultation were
faint and difficult to interpret, and this procedure had limited application.

Another diagnostic method for evaluating chest diseases in the

31

pre-stethoscope era was percussion, the technique of tapping the chest wall with the fingers. This was described in the last half of the nineteenth century by the Austrian physician Joseph Leopold Auenbrugger (1722–1809), as noted in the opening words to his book *Inventum novum ex percussione thoracis humani, ut signo, abstrusos interni pectoris morbos detegendi*:

> I here present the reader with a new sign which I have discovered for detecting diseases of the chest. This consists in the percussion of the human thorax, whereby, according to the character of the particular sounds thence elicited, an opinion is formed of the internal state of that cavity [1761, p. 123].

Auenbrugger was an accomplished musician and had sufficient talent to be the librettist for Antonio Salieri's opera "The Chimney Sweep." It is thus not surprising that he used musically oriented or suggestive terms in describing his clinical observations: "The sound thus elicited . . . from the healthy chest [when struck] resembles the stifled sound of a drum covered with a thick woollen cloth or other envelope" (1761, p. 125), and "if it yields only a sound like that of a fleshy limb when struck,—disease exists in that region" (1761, p. 128).

Although this work enabled physicians to make more precise diagnoses, it was largely ignored for many years. Finally, shortly before Auenbrugger died, the well-known and influential Jean Nicolas Corvisart, personal physician to Napoleon Bonaparte, published a translated and expanded version of Auenbrugger's book, giving full credit to the originator of this valuable procedure.

One of Corvisart's most famous pupils, René Théophile Hyacinthe Laënnec, became particularly interested in chest diseases. In 1819, the art of physical diagnosis was revolutionized by Laënnec's epoch-making publication of the famous *Traité de l'auscultation médiate*. Perhaps the excitement and significance of the occasion when this new method of examination was first used can best be appreciated in re-reading the author's words as translated by John Forbes in the first American edition of this book, entitled *A Treatise on the Diseases of the Chest*, published four years later:

> In 1816, I was consulted by a young woman labouring under general symptoms of diseased heart, and in whose case percussion and the application of the hand were of little avail on account of the great degree of fatness. The other method just mentioned being rendered inadmissible by the age and sex

of the patient [application of the ear to the chest], I happened to recollect a simple and well-known fact in acoustics, and fancied, at the same time, that it might be turned to some use on the present occasion. The fact I allude to is the augmented impression of sound when conveyed through certain solid bodies,—as when we hear the scratch of a pin at one end of a piece of wood, on applying our ear to the other. Immediately, on this suggestion, I rolled a quire of paper into a sort of cylinder and applied one end of it to the region of the heart and the other to my ear, and was not a little surprised and pleased, to find that I could thereby perceive the action of the heart in a manner much more clear and distinct than I had ever been able to do by the immediate application of the ear. From this moment I imagined that the circumstance might furnish means for enabling us to ascertain the character, not only of the action of the heart, but of every species of sound produced by the motion of all the thoracic viscera. With this conviction, I forthwith commenced at the Hospital Necker a series of observations, which has been continued to the present time. The result has been, that I have been enabled to discover a set of new signs of diseases of the chest, for the most part certain, simple, and prominent, and calculated, perhaps, to render the diagnosis of the diseases of the lungs, heart and pleura, as decided and circumstantial, as the indications furnished to the surgeon by the introduction of the finger or sound, in the complaints wherein these are used [1819, pp. 211–212].

With the invention of the stethoscope (a combined form of two Greek words meaning to look at the chest), the moral dilemma of whether or not to place the ear directly upon the female chest was avoided by inserting a "mediator," the stethoscope, between the physician and the patient—hence, the term "mediate auscultation" (Comroe, 1983, p. 94). In addition, the new instrument amplified the faint sounds coming from the heart and lungs, improving the ability of physicians to make a correct diagnosis.

On the spur of the moment, Laënnec had made his first instrument of paper rolled into the shape of a cylinder. He soon turned to other materials, finally settling on wood designed so as to transmit sound in the best way possible (Figure 4.1):

It [the instrument] consists simply of a cylinder of wood, perforated in its centre longitudinally, by a bore three lines in diameter, and formed so as to come apart in the middle, for the benefit of being more easily carried. One extremity of the cylinder is hollowed out into the form of a funnel to the depth of an inch and half, which cavity can be obliterated at pleasure by a piece of wood so constructed as to fit it exactly, with the exception of the central bore which is continued through it, so as to render the instrument in all cases, a pervious tube. The complete instrument,—that is, with the funnel-shaped plug infixed,—is used in exploring the signs obtained through the medium of the voice and the action of the heart; the other modification, or with the stopper removed, is for examining the sounds communicated by respiration. . . . This

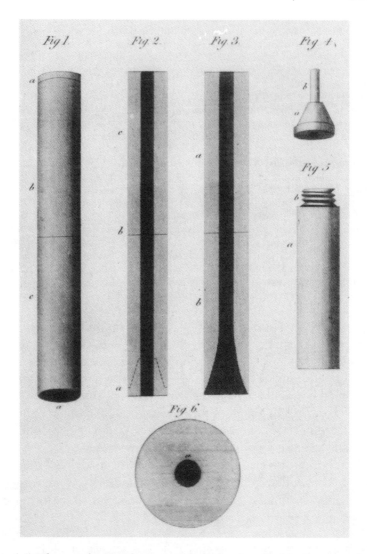

FIG. 4.1. The wooden *Stethoscope* or *Cylinder* described by Laënnec during the early years of the nineteenth century. The three parts of the instrument are pictured fully assembled and after being dismantled, with a longitudinal section demonstrating the central bore or hole running through the entire length. The part labelled *a* in "Fig. 2" was placed on the patient's chest; the opposite end, labelled *c*, was applied to the physician's ear. *Source*: Laënnec, R. T. H. (1819), A *Treatise on the Diseases of the Chest*, tr. J. Forbes. Philadelphia: J. Webster, 1823. Plate VIII. Courtesy of The Library of The Hartford Medical Society, Hartford, CT.

instrument I commonly designate simply the *Cylinder,* sometimes the *Steth-oscope* [Laënnec, 1819, p. 212].

Laënnec was very careful to add that his new method of auscultation should be used together with the method of Auenbrugger, noting specifically that "the latter [percussion] acquires quite a fresh degree of value through the simultaneous employment of the former [auscultation], and becomes applicable in many cases, wherein its solitary employment is either useless or hurtful" (1819, p. 213). Shortly after publication of the second edition of his book in 1826, Laënnec died at the age of 45. He had meticulously correlated the sounds heard through the stethoscope with the pathologic findings at postmortem examination, thus linking the sciences of pathology and physical diagnosis. For this major contribution, he deservedly should be honored as the father of modern clinical medicine.

During the remainder of the nineteenth century, numerous modifications of the stethoscope were developed as its appearance gradually assumed the form familiar to present-day physicians and as the science of acoustics became better understood. The rigid wooden cylinder of the monaural instrument (single ear piece) became narrower, and the ear and chest pieces were modified. By the latter half of the nineteenth century, the introduction of vulcanized rubber allowed the stethoscope to become flexible, a boon to both physician and patient. One of the earliest flexible binaural stethoscopes in common usage, described by George Cammann in the United States (1855), consisted of

an objective end, made of ebony, the extremity of which is about two inches in diameter, two tubes composed of gum elastic and metallic wire, two metallic tubes of German silver, two ivory knobs at the aural extremity, and a movable elastic spring, so arranged as to adjust it, and keep it in its proper position [1855, pp. 140–141].

For many years, there was considerable controversy regarding the technical and acoustic merits of the monaural versus the binaural instrument, the former being preferred by many well into the twentieth century prior to general acceptance of the binaural design (Figure 4.2a,b).

Information on Laënnec's new instrument and on its diagnostic capabilities was disseminated rapidly during the ninteenth century through the writings of many physicians—John Forbes in his previously mentioned English translation of Laënnec's monograph, *An*

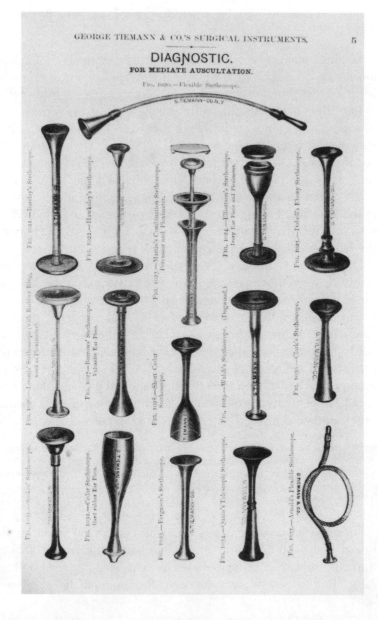

FIG. 4.2. A variety of designs for monaural and binaural stethoscopes, known by many different names, as advertised in a late nineteenth-century catalogue of surgical instruments. *Source: The American Armamentarium Chirurgicum,*

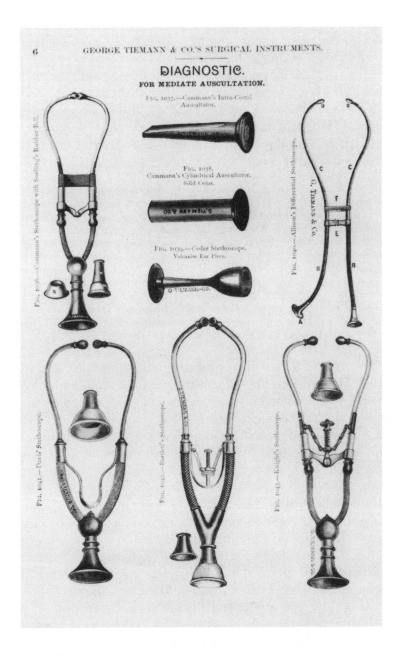

George Tiemann & Co., New York, 1889. Courtesy of the Lyman Maynard Stowe Library, University of Connecticut Health Center, Farmington, CT.

Introduction to the Use of the Stethoscope by William Stokes (1825), the descriptions of murmurs and heart sounds by James Hope in *A Treatise on the Diseases of the Heart and Great Vessels* (1832), and the well-known *The Young Stethoscopist, or the Student's Aid to Auscultation* by Henry Ingersoll Bowditch from Massachusetts, an authority on auscultation. Shortly after it was first described, medical students at Harvard University were introduced to the stethoscope by James Jackson, a leading physician at the Massachusetts General Hospital, who had this to say:

> The use of the *stethoscope* is founded on the following circumstances. The motion of the air in the lungs, with all the obstacles to the regular passage of it, is productive of sounds, which may be heard by placing the ear on the chest. So also are the motions of the heart capable of being ascertained by the ear. But these sounds in the thorax may be ascertained most conveniently through a cylinder of wood, or of other material; one end of the instrument being rested on the chest, and one end being applied to the ear. When such an instrument is used the auscultation is mediate; when the ear is applied to the thorax the auscultation is immediate. If the instrument be applied when the patient is speaking, a tremor is perceived over healthy lungs; but when the lungs are diseased, or compressed, the changes are manifested by certain peculiar changes in the sounds transmitted through the instrument [1827, pp. 52–53].

The use of the stethoscope rapidly gave birth to new diagnostic findings. Many of these are still remembered in present-day cardiology textbooks with eponymous designations indicating the name of the physician making the original observation. Two of the best known of these, particularly to generations of medical students and cardiologists, are the Austin Flint and the Graham Steell murmurs. The former, an apical diastolic murmur that mimics the murmur of organic mitral stenosis, was described by Flint as "a mitral direct murmur . . . [that] may exist without mitral contraction and without any mitral lesions, provided there be aortic lesions involving considerable aortic regurgitation" (1862, p. 53). The functional murmur of pulmonic regurgitation in patients with mitral stenosis or severe pulmonary hypertension, the Graham Steell murmer, was described in an article entitled "The murmur of high-pressure in the pulmonary artery" (Steell, 1888).

Medical wit and humor could hardly resist the opportunity presented by this instrument. In a poem entitled "The Stethoscope Song," Oliver Wendell Holmes, writer-physician and Professor of Anatomy and Physiology at Harvard during the nineteenth century, described the erroneous diagnoses that resulted when strange noises made by two flies trapped within a stethoscope were misinterpreted by a young physician as signifying disease. At the same time, Holmes ridiculed the pompous medical terminology used in recording these and other clinical observations. The poem ends with the thought that doctors should rely on their own senses as well as new technology, a message still relevant today:

> Now use your ears, all that you can,
>   But don't forget to mind your eyes,
> Or you may be cheated, like this young man,
>   By a couple of silly, abnormal flies [1849, p. 263].

Laënnec devised the stethoscope in an effort to distance himself from a female patient so as to avoid the embarrassment of placing his own ear directly upon her chest during a physical examination, then the accepted procedure for listening to sounds within the thorax. In the present era, however, in which sophisticated medical instrumentation and testing has at times fostered a physical and emotional detachment of physician and patient, the stethoscope, whatever its other attributes, may serve to bring the two closer together. Perhaps the following amusing but pointed comments by Dickinson Richards (1895–1973), a clinician, teacher, and exemplar of the physician engaged in cardiopulmonary research, provide a fitting present-day tribute to an instrument that for so long has faithfully served the medical profession:

Let us pause for a moment and contemplate this humble little device, the stethoscope, by and for itself. Look at it as it hangs on its hook, with its ears up and its rubber legs twisted. Has anyone ever commented how remarkably in this posture it simulates the snakes of the caduceus, the symbol of our old friend Aesculapius? Well, one can say that in this particular posture it is indeed equally symbolic, and equally useless with the Aesculapian wand. Now take it off its hook and slip it deftly in the white coat pocket. It is still no better, still a useless symbol, no matter how portentous the prestige that may happen to stuff out the white coat.

But now suppose we put the thing into operation. There occurs a metamorphosis. I should like to advance the proposition that now this ancient and outdated instrument of nickel, rubber, and plastic has one attribute that transcends all the laboratories that ever were or ever will be built. In order for the stethoscope to function, two things have to happen. *There has to be, by God, a sick man at one end of it and a doctor at the other!* The doctor has to be within thirty inches of his patient. . . .

It might not be too presumptuous to suppose that in being this close to his patient, the doctor might hear, see, feel, or otherwise apprehend something more beyond the momentary lub-dup [sounds] in the earpiece [1962, pp. 7–8].

5

The Recognition of Fever: From the Hand to the Clinical Thermometer

I don't like it; it's a bad sign first to sweat and then
to shiver!

[Plautus, c. 200 B.C., p. 75]

FEVER has long been recognized as a sign of illness. Physicians have also been aware that specific patterns of fever could be related to prognosis, an observation made over 2,000 years ago by Hippocrates and recorded in the work *Of the Epidemics*:

> Fevers are,—the continual, some of which hold during the day and have a remission at night, and others hold during the night and have a remission during the day; semi-tertians, tertians, quartans, quintans, septans, nonans. The most acute, strongest, most dangerous, and fatal diseases, occur in the continual fever. The least dangerous of all, and the mildest and most protracted, is the quartan, for it is not only such from itself, but it also carries off other great diseases. . . . The true tertian comes quickly to a crisis, and is not fatal; but the quintan is the worst of all, for it proves fatal when it precedes an attack of phthisis, and when it supervenes on persons who are already consumptive [c. 400 B.C.a, pp. 368–369].

Perhaps one of the earliest attempts at quantifying and standardizing temperature measurements was made by Galen (131–200 A.D.), using a crude scale based upon the hottest and coldest of known materials—boiling water and ice, respectively—and upon a neutral

41

point as represented by an equal mixture of the two (Taylor, 1942, pp. 129–130). However, the multiple sources of error in this approach made these observations inconstant and of little value. For many years no useful instruments were available for recording body temperature, and the presence of fever could be inferred only from a patient's subjective sensations and appearance, or with the use of a physician's educated hand. Indeed, until the latter half of the nineteenth century, a standardized technique of hand-thermometry was still being carefully taught to medical students of the day, particularly for recognizing regional temperature changes, applying methods that were probably little modified from those used by generations of physicians before them:

> The hand is a thermometer that rich or poor, educated or ignorant, we cannot help carrying with us anywhere. It gives—besides an idea of the temperature rendered more and more accurate by education—a knowledge of the concomitant properties of the parts under exploration, as tension, dryness, etc. [Seguin, 1876, p. 253].

Further on in the same text, Seguin described the actual procedure of taking the temperature using this technique:

> The flat of one or more fingers, or of the whole hand—according to the size and configuration of the surface to be explored—remains hovering a while above and near, to perceive the heat exhaled therefrom; then enters upon a slight contact with this surface to receive the impression of its most superficial temperature; then by a firmer pressure receives the full impression of the skin's temperature; then by gradually deeper pressures acquires the impressions of deeper and deeper seated combustions. Every one of these pressures should be made separately, after the impression of the former has distinctly reached the mind through the inquiring hand. Then the hand is gradually and slowly removed, in order to appreciate these different modifications of temperature in inverse progression, or rather in retrogression [1876, p. 255].

Air, alcohol, and mercury-type thermometers were invented during the seventeenth and eighteenth centuries, with contributions to this field being made by Cornelius Drebbel from Holland (1572–1633), Robert Fludd of St. Johns College, Oxford (1574–1637), and the Italian physicist and astronomer Galileo (1.564–1642). The first medical use of a thermometer has usually been attributed to Santorio Santorio, called Sanctorius (1561–1636), a professor of medicine at the University of Padua, and one of the first physicians to employ precise instruments and quantitative procedures in his work (Figure 5.1). Sanc-

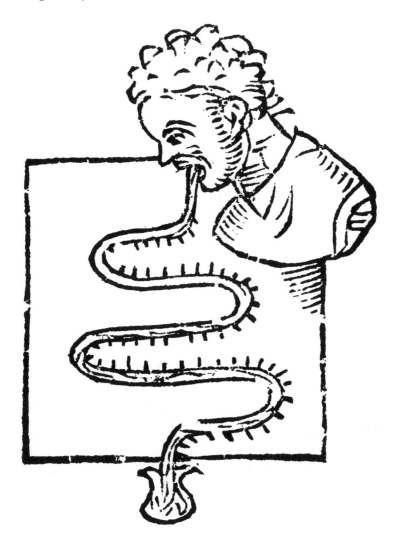

FIG. 5.1. The first illustration of an oral thermometer, devised by Santorio Santorio (Sanctorius) of Padua, and published in 1646 in his *Commentaria in primam fen primi libri Canonis Avicennae*. *Source*: Courtesy of the National Library of Medicine, History of Medicine Division, Bethesda, MD.

torius constructed an instrument made of a thin glass tube, one end of which was shaped into a closed bulb. The other end remained open in order to allow a colored liquid into which it was dipped access to the inside of the tube. Writing in 1612 about his experiences with this instrument, Sanctorius stated in Part III of his *Commentaria in artem Medicinalem Galenis*:

> I must inform you of a marvellous method, by which, with the aid of a glass instrument, I am wont to measure the cold or hot temperature of the air, of all districts, all places and all parts of the body, and so exactly that at any time of the day I can measure with the compass the degrees and ultimate stations of heat and cold [Taylor, 1942, p. 135].

Patients either clamped the closed bulb of the glass tube in their hands or held it in their mouths. As the air within the tube expanded or contracted in response to the temperature of the organ with which it was in contact, the level of the colored liquid entering through the open end of the tube would rise or fall, thus, as Sanctorius indicated, providing an estimate of the temperature of "all places and all parts of the body" (Taylor, 1942, p. 135). Unfortunately, this early thermometer not only measured temperature, but, being exposed to air at one end, also reacted to variations in barometric pressure.

As additional improvements were made, and with the development of standardized scales by Daniel Gabriel Fahrenheit and Anders Celsius (the centigrade scale) during the first half of the eighteenth century, physicians slowly began to realize the benefits to be derived from the thermometer. In 1740, George Martine, trained at the Universities of Edinburgh and Leiden, published some of the first accurate observations of the temperature of healthy people and animals in his *Essays Medical and Philosophical* (Haller, 1985, p. 109). A few years later, Gerhard van Swieten, professor of medicine at the University of Vienna, recommended the mercurial thermometer, writing in his *Commentaries Upon the Aphorisms of Dr. Hermann Boerhaave*:

> When such a thermometer, first used on a healthy man, and marked accordingly on the scale, is either held in the hand of a fever patient, or the bulb placed in his mouth, or laid on his bare chest, or in his axillae . . . the ascent of the mercury to different elevations will show how far the fever heat exceeds the natural and healthy [Haller, 1985, pp. 108–109].

Anton de Haen, a contemporary of van Swieten's in Vienna, extended these observations to the bedside of the patient where, according to Haller, he taught "that the only safe way to determine fever lay in the use of the thermometer. No longer would a physician's touch or the patient's perception be adequate" (1985, p. 109). Further observations were made by James Currie during the course of experiments designed to evaluate the effects of warm and cold water, opium, inanition, and alcohol upon body temperature:

> In taking the heat of the patient, I have generally used a small mercurial thermometer of great sensibility, with a moveable scale, made for me by Mr. Ramsden, after a form invented by the late Mr. Hunter, and used by him in his experiments on the heat of animals, and I have introduced the bulb under the tongue with the lips close, or under the axilla, indifferently; having found by repeated experiments, that the heat in these two places corresponds exactly, and gives a just indication of the heat of the surface of the body [1804, p. 35].

In spite of these reports, use of the thermometer was sporadic, and widespread clinical acceptance of the instrument had to await both technical and practical improvements in its design, and a greater understanding of the significance that temperature measurements had in the clinical diagnosis, prognosis, and treatment of patients. The latter information was provided by Dr. Carl Wunderlich, professor of medicine at Leipzig University, in his classic and masterful book *Das Verhalten der Eigenwärme in Krankheiten* published in 1868, the English edition of which appeared three years later entitled *On the Temperature in Diseases: A Manual of Medical Thermometry*. Relying upon serial temperature recordings in thousands of patients, Wunderlich established two basic facts—*"the constancy of temperature in healthy persons"* and *"the variation of temperature in disease"* (1868, p. 1). Wunderlich was able to describe the specific fluctuations of temperature present in such febrile diseases as typhus, measles, pneumonia, trichinosis, osteomyelitis, and the like, information of considerable diagnostic importance to the physician in an era in which more refined laboratory tests were unavailable. The significance of Wunderlich's observations was immediately recognized, and a plethora of reports describing the temperature changes in many other disorders soon appeared. As stated by Garrison, "He [Wunderlich] found fever a disease and left it a symptom" (1929, p. 431).

One of the earliest clinical thermometers in England was made in the mid-nineteenth century by the instrument maker Louis P. Casella, under the direction of Dr. Aitken of the Royal Victoria Hospital in Netley (Casella, 1869). Although accurate, this instrument had practical disadvantages which made its application difficult, as summarized picturesquely by the well-known English physician, T. Lauder Brunton:

> When I entered upon my duties as house physician [1866–1867] I found, amongst other apparatus for use in the ward, a case containing two clinical thermometers, one straight and the other somewhat bent. Each was about ten inches or more in length and took about five minutes or more to reach the temperature of the body when it was placed in the axilla. This thermometer case I used to carry under my arm as one might carry a gun, and most of the thermometric readings I took myself, rarely entrusting the thermometers to the clinical clerks. The thermometers were known as Aitken's thermometers in the hospital. The clumsy character of these thermometers and the long time they took to rise prevented them from coming into general use [1916, p. 317].

An additional view of this new instrument was given by Samuel Wilks at Guy's Hospital in London in reminiscing about his early years:

> I requested the superintendent at Guy's to procure a clinical thermometer. This he did; it was at the service of any one who might wish to make use of it. I think it was nearly a foot long, and was so great a novelty that it was taken to a South-Eastern meeting of the British Medical Association for exhibition, where the members regarded it with much curiosity and interest although, I am sorry to say, one or two with ridicule [Wilks, 1903, p. 1059].

Dr. T. Clifford Allbutt, commenting that such instruments "are, however, too cumbrous for general practice, and for this reason the thermometer long remained a stranger to the busy practitioner" (1870, p. 437), introduced into medical practice a smaller portable mercury thermometer made by Messrs. Harvey and Reynolds, the prototype of the instrument still in clinical use today.

While these events were taking place in Europe, American physicians were also being introduced to the benefits and advantages of clinical thermometry. Austin Flint in New York wrote:

> Hitherto, in this country [America], the thermometer has been but little used in medical investigations, owing, probably, to a prudential reserve with regard to novelties. Many, however, are now interested in confirming, by personal observation, the correctness of what has been set forth in publications on the other side of the Atlantic. . . .
>
> The use of the thermometer is essential for obtaining accurate, reliable information of the temperature of the body. The information obtained by

merely placing the hand on the body of the patient is inaccurate and unreliable [1866, pp. 81–82].

Edouard Seguin, born and educated in France, came to the United States during the mid-nineteenth century. He became an enthusiastic proponent of medical thermometry, encouraging its use not only by physicians but also by the public at large. In addition, in order to follow and understand the course of a disease, Seguin urged that the temperature be charted in graphic form along with other vital signs, a procedure now uniformly followed in all hospitals:

> But clinical thermometry is never practiced alone. On the contrary, it is supported by the study of other symptoms, and its indications are mostly collected with those given by the pulse-beats and the breathing; forming in their ensemble and continuity "the record of the three great vital signs."
> This triple observation necessitates the formation of a diagram (in itself an important instrument of diagnosis), upon which the rise and fall of the vital signs are not only recorded daily, but connected from morning to night by curves or lines. This triple track of diseases may be seen illustrated in German and English publications [1866–1867, p. 518].

Thus, over 100 years ago, physicians had available to them a reliable and useful instrument that served an important diagnostic and prognostic purpose. The benefit of a careful recording of a patient's temperature, although now surrounded by a myriad of other objective data, has not diminished over the years.

6

Measurement of Blood Pressure

STEPHEN Hales, an ordained minister and a scientist in eighteenth-century England, wrote a letter "To the King's Most Excellent Majesty" that may well exemplify the spirit and purpose of all those who have engaged in scientific pursuits throughout the age, saying in part:

> The study of nature will ever yield us fresh matter of entertainment, and we have great reason to bless God, for the faculties and abilities he has given us, and the strong desire he has implanted in our minds, to search into and contemplate his works, in which the farther we go, the more we see the signatures of his wisdom and power, every thing pleases and instructs us, because in every thing we see a wise design.
>
> As the beautiful fabric of this world was chiefly framed for and adapted to the use of man, so the greater insight we get into the nature and properties of things, so much the more beneficial will they be to us, the more will our real riches thereby increase, the more also will man's original grant of dominion over the creatures be inlarged [sic] [Hales, 1733, pp. A3–A4].

Qualitative assessment of the pulse by palpation has been performed by physicians since early Egyptian times. However, it was not until the experiments of Hales that blood pressure and pulse pressure were measured for the first time. These studies, introduced by the above letter to the King and published under the title of *Statical Essays: Containing Haemastatics*, contain the following much-quoted description:

> In December I caused a *mare* to be tied down alive on her back; she was 14 hands high, and about 14 years of age, had a fistula on her withers, was neither very lean nor yet lusty: having laid open the left crural artery about 3 inches from her belly, I inserted into it a brass pipe whose bore was 1/6 of an

inch in diameter; and to that, by means of another brass pipe which was fitly adapted to it, I fixed a glass tube, of nearly the same diameter, which was 9 feet in length: then untying the ligature on the artery, the blood rose in the tube 8 feet 3 inches perpendicular above the level of the left ventricle of the heart: but it did not attain to its full height at once; it rushed up about half way in an instant, and afterwards gradually at each pulse 12, 8, 6, 4, 2, and sometimes 1 inch: when it was at its full height, it would rise and fall at and after each pulse 2, 3, or 4 inches [Hales, 1733, pp. 1–2].[1]

In 1828, nearly one hundred years later, the Frenchman Jean Marie Poiseuille improved upon this unwieldy procedure by substituting a less cumbersome mercury manometer for the long glass tube previously used by Hales, attaching the instrument to a cannula filled with potassium carbonate to prevent blood from clotting (Booth, 1977, pp. 794–795). The cannula was inserted directly into arteries of experimental animals, with pressures determined in blood vessels as small as two millimeters in diameter. A few years later, Carl Ludwig (1847) modified Poiseuille's equipment by placing a float with an attached pen upon the open mercury column, positioned so as to allow the pen to write upon a revolving cylindrical drum called a kymograph or wave writer (Booth, 1977, p. 795). Movements of the vertical mercury column responding to changes in blood pressure could thus be accurately recorded. The contributions of Bernard, Chauveau, and Marey during the mid-nineteenth century to the measurement of pressure within the heart have been noted in another chapter.

The first direct peripheral blood pressure measurement in a human being was made by Jean Faivre (1856) during an operation by connecting an artery to a mercury manometer. It is of interest for those presently involved in surgery or intensive care medicine to note that determining blood pressure by inserting a cannula directly into an artery preceded by many years the development of a noninvasive or indirect procedure.

In the mid-nineteenth century, Karl Vierordt postulated that by measuring the counterpressure necessary to obliterate the pulsation in an artery, it might be possible to record blood pressure indirectly without puncturing the vessel (Booth, 1977, pp. 795–796). His instrument was improved upon by Marey. To use this apparatus, the patient's arm was placed in a water-filled glass chamber and connected

[1]For ease of reading, the old English spelling used by Hales in this and the preceding citation has been changed by the author into the modern form.

to a sphygmograph to register its arterial pulsations. By altering the pressure of the water within the glass chamber, excursions of the arterial pulsations could be changed, with the pressure level at which no further movements were recorded determining the systolic blood pressure. Although considered ingenious, the device was too cumbersome and unwieldy for clinical application (Major, 1930, pp. 52–53).

During the 1880s, Samuel Siegfried Ritter von Basch, professor of medicine in Vienna, made an instrument that was to evolve in later years into the modern sphygmomanometer. The edges of a water-filled rubber bag were drawn up securely around a bulb that formed the end of a mercury-containing tube or manometer. This arrangement caused changes of pressure in the rubber bag to be transmitted to the mercury column, which would accordingly rise or fall in the tube. The water-filled bag was pressed over an arterial pulse with increasing intensity or force until the pulsations beyond the site of its application disappeared. At that point, the height of the mercury column would be recorded as the systolic pressure. Further modifications of this instrument over the following years included the use of an aneroid rather than a mercury manometer (Booth, 1977; Lawrence, 1979).

It was not, however, until the work of Scipione Riva-Rocci from Italy appeared in 1896 in a report entitled "Un nuovo sfigmomanometro" that a clinically useful noninvasive method for determining blood pressure became available, one that remains the basis of the present-day technique and is familiar to all in medicine. As summarized by Lewis (1941) and Booth (1977), Riva-Rocci wrapped a distensible rubber bag or cuff around the entire circumference of an arm so that when the bag was inflated by means of a rubber bulb, there was equal compression applied to the arm from all sides as the radial pulse was obliterated. The pressure within the cuff was registered by an attached mercury manometer. As the pressure within the inflated cuff was lowered, reappearance of the radial pulse could be used to determine the level of the systolic pressure.

This palpatory technique, however, was limited to measuring the systolic pressure. In order to accurately determine both systolic and diastolic pressures, physicians began to examine more closely the oscillations transmitted from the compressed artery to the mercury in the manometer. As the pressure in the cuff was lowered, it was observed that the initial appearance of oscillations in the manometer reflected the systolic level of pressure, whereas the transition from large to small oscillations as the cuff was deflated still further defined the diastolic level. A sensitive-enough instrument with a needle pressure gauge was devised by Hill and Barnard for recording these measurements (1897), a useful advance in making such observations clinically feasible (Figure 6.1).

It remained, however, for a surgeon from Russia, Nikolai S. Korotkov (1874–1920), to describe the final step in the evolution of the techniques for determining blood pressure—the auscultatory method in use today throughout the world. Korotkov's brief but significant presentation was made at a meeting of the Imperial Military Medical Academy of St. Petersburg and reported in a bulletin from the Academy:

> On the basis of his observations the speaker [Korotkov] has come to the conclusion, that the completely compressed artery under normal circumstances does not produce any sounds. Utilizing this phenomenon he proposes the auditory method of determining the blood pressure in man. The cuff of Riva-Rocci is placed on the middle third of the upper arm, the pressure within the cuff is quickly raised up to the complete cessation of circulation below the cuff. Then, letting the mercury of the manometer fall, one listens to the artery just below the cuff with a children's stethoscope. At first, no sounds are heard. With the falling of the mercury in the manometer, down to a certain height, the first short tones appear; their appearance indicates the passage of part of the pulse wave under the cuff. It follows that the manometric figure at which the first tone appears corresponds to the maximal pressure. With the further fall of the mercury in the manometer the systolic compression murmurs are heard, which pass again into tones (second). Finally all sounds disappear. The time of the cessation of sounds indicates the free passage of the pulse wave; in other words, at the moment of the disappearance of the sounds, the minimal blood pressure within the artery preponderates over the pressure in the cuff. Consequently, the manometric figures at this time correspond to the minimal blood pressure. Experiments on animals gave confirmative results. The first sound-tones appear (10 to 12 mm.) earlier than the pulse, for the palpation of which (e.g., in the radial artery) the inrush of the greater part of the pulse wave is required [1905, pp. 127–128].

Thus the famous Korotkov (or Korotkoff) sounds for determining both the systolic and the diastolic pressure made their debut into medical practice. Clinical sphygmomanometry was born. The advantages of this method for determining blood pressure were soon recognized, as noted by McWilliam and Melvin a few years later:

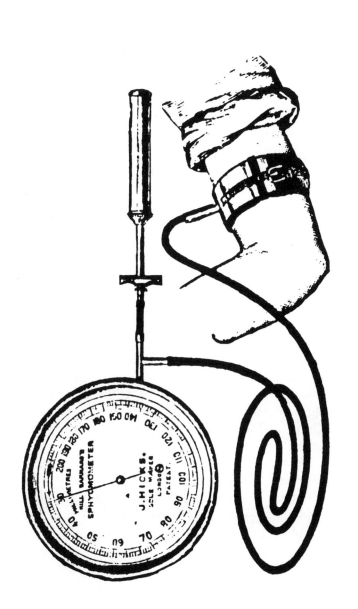

FIG. 6.1. A blood pressure recording instrument designed by Hill and Barnard (1897) in the late nineteenth century, an early approach toward making such measurements more accurate and clinically useful. *Source:* Hill, L., & Barnard, H. (1897), A simple and accurate form of sphygmometer or arterial pressure gauge contrived for clinical use. *Brit. Med. J.*, 2:904.

The simplicity, ease, and rapidity of this method [auditory] are strong points in its favour. It gives all the information that is to be obtained by more cumbrous and time-consuming methods, and that with greater precision, the index being a much sharper one than is present in other methods. . . . It is greatly superior to the palpatory and sphygmographic methods that have been proposed. We are satisfied that all the evidence as to diastolic pressure gained by the other methods, and much more also, can be better obtained by the quick and simple auditory method. The diastolic estimation in this way is as easy as that of systolic pressure, and is relatively little, if at all, complicated by certain sources of fallacy (for example, state of arterial wall) which may come into question in systolic estimation.

This method, measuring the diastolic as well as the systolic pressure, has the great advantage, as compared with the ordinary tactile method, of giving the numerical range of pressure variation in the artery during the whole cycle of the pulse beat, that is, the pulse pressure range [1914, p. 697].

Over a period of two centuries, an international group of investigators made significant contributions to the development of a universally accepted procedure that has allowed one of the most pervasive cardiovascular diseases of Western civilization—hypertension—to be easily recognized and, as such, to be accessible to the benefits of modern therapies. The simplicity with which a blood pressure determination can now be made has enabled large epidemiologic studies to be conducted in order to evaluate the prognosis of different levels of pressure and in order to observe the results of appropriate therapy. Recognition of an elevated blood pressure (hypertension) is the first step in an examination to distinguish patients with secondary hypertension due to known causes, such as coarctation of the aorta, renal disease, and pheochromocytoma, from those with essential or primary hypertension, which has no known cause. Significant segments of the population can be easily and economically screened for hypertension, and if treatment is needed, blood pressure monitoring, many times by patients themselves, can be readily performed. Because of its great value, this instrument must be placed alongside the stethoscope, thermometer, and hypodermic syringe as a major contribution to the modern-day practice of medicine.

7

The Electrocardiograph:
Recording the Heart's Electricity

An instrument of precision has been placed at our command.
[Lewis, 1915, p. 37]

MORE than two thousand years ago, Aristotle, in a treatise entitled *Historia animalium (History of animals)*, described electricity in a living creature:

The torpedo [fish] narcotizes the creatures that it wants to catch, overpowering them by the power of shock that is resident in its body, and feeds upon them; it also hides in the sand and mud, and catches all the creatures that swim in its way and come under its narcotizing influence. This phenomenon has been actually observed in operation. The sting-ray also conceals itself, but not exactly in the same way. That the creatures get their living by this means is obvious from the fact that, whereas they are peculiarly inactive, they are often caught with mullets in their interior, the swiftest of fishes. . . . [T]he torpedo is known to cause a numbness even in human beings [n.d., p. 146].

It was not until the eighteenth and nineteenth centuries that important progress was made in understanding and in recording these electrical forces within living tissue. In the late eighteenth century, Luigi Galvani, professor of anatomy at the University of Bologna, observed that the hind limbs of a dissected frog contracted upon electrical stimulation. The sequence of events leading to this discovery, and the excitement and enthusiasm of the moment, can best be appreciated by referring to Galvani's description of the occasion:

> The course of the work has progressed in the following way. I dissected a frog and prepared it. . . . Having in mind other things, I placed the frog on the same table as an electrical machine . . . so that the animal was completely separated from and removed at a considerable distance from the machine's conductor. When one of my assistants by chance lightly applied the point of a scalpel to the inner crural nerves . . . suddenly all the muscles of the limbs were seen so to contract that they appeared to have fallen into violent tonic convulsions. Another assistant who was present when we were performing electrical experiments thought he observed that this phenomenon occurred when a spark was discharged from the conductor of the electrical machine. . . . Marvelling at this, he immediately brought the unusual phenomenon to my attention when I was completely engrossed and contemplating other things. Hereupon I became extremely enthusiastic and eager to repeat the experiment so as to clarify the obscure phenomenon and make it known. I myself, therefore, applied the point of the scalpel first to one then to the other crural nerve, while at the same time some one of the assistants produced a spark; the phenomenon repeated itself in precisely the same manner as before. Violent contractions were induced in the individual muscles of the limbs and the prepared animal reacted just as though it were seized with tetanus at the very moment when the sparks were discharged [1791, pp. 45–47].

Almost fifty years later, Carlo Matteucci at the University of Pisa observed that the muscle of a nerve–muscle preparation will contract if the attached nerve is placed across another contracting or stimulated muscle (Burch and DePasquale, 1964, p. 22). This experimental work of the 1840s was extended a few years later by Kölliker and Müller, who placed a similar nerve–muscle preparation on the surface of a beating heart, noting that the muscle was stimulated with every systolic contraction of the heart. Thus, by using the frog nerve–muscle preparation as a galvanometer, the electric potential of heart muscle could be demonstrated (Katz and Hellerstein, 1964, pp. 283–284).

Early galvanometers or recording devices capable of measuring electric currents in the heart were relatively insensitive, despite important progress made by Du Bois-Reymond and his pupil Julius Bernstein in developing the rheotome and differential rheotome, and despite the classic experiments of Burdon-Sanderson and Page in England. The latter investigators, using the rheotome to evaluate the order of the excitation in the ventricles of a heart of a frog, demonstrated that "1. Every excited part of the surface of the ventricle is during the excitatory state *negative* to every unexcited part. 2. The excitatory state is propagated in all directions" [1880, p. 426]. In 1875, Gabriel Lippmann, later a Nobel prize recipient in physics, devised the mercury capillary electrometer, a more versatile and sensitive instrument that replaced the rheotome for measuring bioelectric currents (Katz and Hellerstein, 1964, pp. 287–289). Its design was based on the principle that surface tension at the junction of mercury and dilute sulfuric acid varies when the electric potential difference between the two substances is altered. Movements of the mercury meniscus between the two solutions were then magnified and recorded. With this instrument, Augustus Désiré Waller, a physiologist at London University, demonstrated for the first time that variations in electrical potential from the human heart could be obtained from the surface of the body. These historically significant recordings were described by Waller as follows:

> If a pair of electrodes (zinc covered by chamois leather and moistened with brine) are strapped to the front and back of the chest, and connected with a Lippmann's capillary electrometer, the mercury in the latter will be seen to move slightly but sharply at each beat of the heart. If the movements of the column of mercury are photographed on a travelling plate simultaneously with those of an ordinary cardiographic lever a record is obtained. . . . Each beat of the heart is seen to be accompanied by an electrical variation [1887, p. 229].

It is of additional interest that Waller used chest leads in these experiments in order to place the electrodes as near as possible to the source of the electricity—the heart. Although this instrument was more sensitive than those used earlier, its movements were sluggish and inexact, owing to the inertia of the mercury.

Willem Einthoven (1860–1927) of Leiden University in Holland, dissatisfied with previous attempts at measuring and examining cardiac potentials, devised his own simpler but more sensitive and accurate galvanometer:

> This instrument—the string galvanometer—is essentially composed of a thin silver-coated quartz filament, which is stretched like a string, in a strong magnetic field. When an electric current is conducted through this quartz filament, the filament reveals a movement which can be observed and photographed by means of considerable magnification. . . . It is possible to regulate the sensitivity of the galvanometer very accurately within broad limits by tightening or loosening the string [1903, p. 723].

Einthoven's first electrocardiograph weighed 600 pounds and required five people to operate (Burch and DePasquale, 1964, p. 114). The success of the instrument, however, and the high quality of the tracings it produced prompted commercial interest on the part of Edelmann and Sons of Munich. Indeed, their machine, a model of which was brought to the United States in 1909 by Alfred Cohn, then at Mount Sinai Hospital in New York, was said to be the first electrocardiograph in the Western Hemisphere (Burch and DePasquale, 1964, pp. 35–36). Because of a dispute over royalties, Einthoven later turned to the Cambridge Scientific Instrument Company, Ltd., of London to redesign, manufacture, and market his instrument under the direction of W. D. Duddell (Figure 7.1). One of the early units made by this company was installed at the University College Hospital in London for Sir Thomas Lewis, a pioneer in the clinical use of this new procedure (Burch and DePasquale, 1964, p. 33).

A series of significant studies was performed by Einthoven in the years that followed, establishing the diagnostic capabilities of the new instrument and demonstrating examples of abnormal electrocardiographic tracings in disease states. Some of this work was reviewed at a meeting in London of the Chelsea Clinical Society on March 19, 1912, in which Einthoven clearly indicated many of the fundamentals of basic electrocardiography as well as the future direction of this field:

> The application of the electrocardiography to clinical examination gives valuable data in two different ways. In the first place, it shows the time relations between the action of the ventricles and the auricles. The difference in time between the contraction of these two parts of the heart can be measured easily and accurately. Diseases such as Stokes-Adams's, in which the auricles have a rhythm different from that of the ventricles, and which sometimes give difficulties when examined by the older methods, are always immediately recognised, electrocardiographically. And further may be mentioned that a new insight has been obtained into several other diseases, among which auricular fibrillation takes a prominent place.
>
> But this evening we shall pass over this first group of symptoms, and we shall limit our attention to the second one, which is concerned with the form of the EKG. If this form is perfect, it must be the exact expression of the changes in potential difference which take place between two parts of the human body. It is self evident that a perfect form can only be obtained by means of a perfect instrument, and it need not be mentioned that such an instrument does not exist. The capillary electrometer is not rapid enough when made sufficiently sensitive, and therefore not suitable for clinical purposes. The oscillograph suffers from the same fault, although in a less degree, and has, moreover, the great disadvantage that the movements of the recording mirror are oscillatory. On the contrary, the string galvanometer is in general

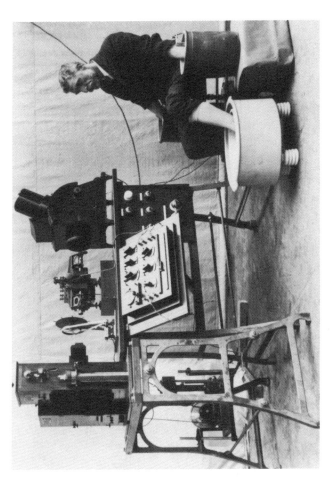

FIG. 7.1. Original Cambridge electrocardiograph of 1912, produced under agreement with Willem Einthoven, the father of electrocardiography. The instrument was large, with electrodes consisting of cylinders or jars containing electrolyte solutions into which the arms and legs of the patient were placed. Strap-on electrodes similar to those in current use did not make their appearance until several years later. *Source:* Courtesy of Cambridge Medical Instruments, Ossining, NY.

sufficient for clinical purposes, and by means of this instrument we are able to approximate the exact form of the EKG so closely that the remaining divergences from it become practically imperceptible [1912, p. 853].

At this meeting, Einthoven explained an important concept relating the forms of the complexes in the limb leads to each other:

> From the nature of the case there must be a connexion between the curves obtained by the three different leads from the same person. If two forms are known, the third may be calculated from them. The difference between the electrical tensions of leads I and II must be equal to the electrical tension of lead III. This may be formulated: lead II − lead I = lead III [1912, p. 854].

Einthoven also referred to the U wave of the electrocardiogram, a wave form that even to the present day is incompletely understood, stating that it "may have a considerable height in pathological cases. This wave U is also present in the curves from normal hearts, but in these cases it is very low as a rule. . . . The significance of it and the reason for its inconstancy are for the present not known with surety" (1912, p. 856).

Later in his presentation, Einthoven discussed early concepts of what would eventually be referred to as the Einthoven equilateral triangle:

> The difficulties are solved at once, however, if we apply a schema in which the human body is represented by a plane, homogeneous plate in the form of an equilateral triangle, *RLF*. (Fig. 26.) From its corners the current is lead off to the galvanometer. *R* corresponds to the right and *L* to the left arm, while *F* indicates the potential of both feet. Thus, a lead from *R* and *L* corresponds to lead I, from *R* and *F* to lead II, and from *L* and *F* to lead III. A small spot *H* in the middle of the triangle represents the heart. We assume that in a given moment the potential differences in the heart are so distributed that their resultant takes the direction of the arrow drawn in the figure. This direction indicates the direction of the current in the heart. The angle which the arrow forms with the side *RL* is call *a*. We shall call the angle positive if, when looking towards the front wall of the chest of the patient, the arrow rotates with the hands of the clock; negative if it rotates in the opposite direction [1912, p. 860].

In recognition of his remarkable accomplishments, Einthoven was awarded the 1924 Nobel Prize for Medicine, a truly deserved tribute to the man who is remembered as the father of electrocardiography. The brilliance of his work introduced a fresh perspective and began a new era in the field of clinical cardiology.

Prior to the development of the electrocardiograph, devices known as sphygmographs and polygraphs were used both for examining movements and pulsations of the heart and blood vessels and for evaluating cardiac arrhythmias, with James Mackenzie being one of the leading proponents of these techniques (1910). However, the advantages of Einthoven's new instrument as a means of analyzing irregularities of heart rhythm in clinical practice were quickly recognized by the renowned English cardiologist Sir Thomas Lewis (1881–1945), who noted enthusiastically on a visit to the United States that "an instrument of precision has been placed at our command, an instrument which permits us to record the inner workings [of the heart] and brings us into direct contact with its wheels. This instrument is the string galvanometer of Einthoven" (1915, p. 37).

During the early years of electrocardiography, advances were many and occurred in rapid succession. Sir Thomas Lewis, using Einthoven's instrument to great advantage, performed extensive research, particularly in the area of cardiac arrhythmias. His publications were numerous, with perhaps the following excerpt from one of his articles providing an insightful overview on the subject as seen by one of its greatest pioneers:

> To sum up, galvanometric examination of the heart is important from many points of view. It may give indications of enlargement of the walls of one or other cardiac chamber; it may accurately locate small lesions in the musculature. It informs us when the heart beat starts at the normal impulse centre or away from it; in the last named condition it tells us that the rhythm is no longer under the normal nervous control—a fact which is of fundamental importance in the management of our case; it tells us within certain limits where the new beats have their origin. It gives us a separate record of contraction in auricle and in ventricle, and accurately defines the time relation of contraction in one chamber and the other; thereby it frequently elucidates physical signs which otherwise remain obscure. It provides us with a perfect means of ascertaining the functional efficiency of the auriculo-ventricular bundle, the sole conducting tract upon which the ventricle depends for the reception of impulses which start its contractions. It allows us to differentiate between separate forms of slow and rapid heart action, which are of totally different significance. It provides us with an analysis of every form of cardiac irregularity, an analysis which is unrivalled in its precision by any other method. While the information derived from it relates essentially to the condition of the muscle, the method is often helpful in the diagnosis of lesions of the valves. It brings us into nearer contact with the functions of the heart muscle than does any other clinical method; it is a precise means of studying the heart as a living and moving organ.
>
> The information obtained by electro-cardiography is not, as commonly

thought, of purely scientific interest in the analysis of disordered heart action. It has a great and growing value in the practical management of patients. There are few heart cases in which our knowledge is not added to by its employment, and in a steadily increasing percentage facts which are essential if sound prognosis and treatment are to be attempted are elicited. The time is at hand, if it has not already come, when an examination of the heart is incomplete if this new method is neglected [1912, p. 67].

James and Williams published one of the first articles on electrocardiography to appear in an American medical journal (1910). Fred Smith in Chicago noted the changes in the electrocardiogram that occurred after ligating branches of the coronary arteries in dogs (1918), a change that was also observed by Herrick the following year in a patient with a myocardial infarct (1919). The characteristic T wave abnormality in patients with a myocardial infarction was reported by Pardee (1920), while Wilson and Herrmann (1920) and Fahr (1920) made major contributions to understanding bundle-branch block. Feil and Siegel described

inversion of the S-T portion of the curve in Leads I and II while the patients complained of substernal pain [angina]. . . . The curves resumed their previous contours after the pain subsided. . . .
It is suggested . . . that the changes observed in the S-T portion of the electrocardiogram of the patients now under study, represent transient vascular changes in the heart muscle [1928, p. 260].

The significance of this early study by Feil and Siegel is apparent in light of present-day methods of electrocardiographic monitoring of patients with chest pain in intensive-care units and the importance of stress tests in evaluating the cause of chest symptoms.

Of pivotal interest, particularly as it triggered a host of important discoveries in the years that followed, was the report by Wolff, Parkinson, and White (1930) entitled "Bundle-branch block with short P-R interval in healthy young people prone to paroxysmal tachycardia," the WPW syndrome and the best known of the pre-excitation syndromes.

Present-day electrocardiography, including ambulatory electrocardiography, coronary care unit monitoring, electrophysiological testing, stress testing, surgical ablation of the source of arrhythmias, and their like, all have as their common ancestry the invention of the electrocardiograph by Willem Einthoven. Through his perfection of a machine that could accurately record the electricity of the heart, generations of physicians have been provided with a useful and practical instrument to assist them in diagnosing cardiac disorders.

Section II

Staples of Pharmacology and Other Remedies

THE employment of opium, iron, colchicine, and atropine as therapeutic agents was for many hundreds of years based on folklore and empiricism. However, many keen and critical observations made during this same period eventually led to a more rational understanding of these substances. In retrospect, the high degree of specificity with which our forebears used these preparations without knowledge of basic pharmacology and physiology is indeed amazing.

Examination and measurement of urine have long been traditional functions of the physician or healer, and it is not surprising that diuretic substances of various types have always attracted the attention of the medical profession. These agents, limited as they formerly were in their effectiveness and imperfect as was the knowledge of their mechanisms of action, have a fascinating history that preceded by many years the use of today's potent medications. The development of life-saving therapies for patients with pernicious anemia and diabetes mellitus, vitamin B_{12} and insulin, respectively, was the outgrowth of careful medical detective work that over a period of many years uncovered the pathophysiology of the disease processes involved. Both discoveries were landmarks in medical research and therapeutics. The vast amount of knowledge now available about oxygen, the clarification of its role in the body, and the development of oxygen and inhalation therapy, are tributes to the facile and inquisitive minds of many in-

65

vestigators spanning a period of more then three hundred years, the details of which could fill a book several times over.

To conclude this section, and somewhat distinct from other more traditional medical therapies, the centuries-old and unusual remediable powers attributable to leeches, to music, and to wine are discussed. These three forms of treatment continue to have their present-day advocates for the management of selected clinical disorders.

8

Opium and Morphine: Blessing or Curse?

Thou hast the keys of Paradise, oh, just, subtle, and
mighty opium!
[Thomas De Quincey, 1821]

THROUGHOUT history, opium and morphine have frequently
crossed paths with wars, smugglers, famous people, addicts, literary works, far-away places, the exotic, and the mysterious. Opium,
a name derived from the Greek word "opos" for juice, is obtained by
scarifying or incising the seed capsule of the poppy plant *Papaver
somniferum* and harvesting the milky-white liquid or sap that appears.
The collecting process has changed little over hundreds of years.

Egyptian papyri from 1500 B.C. mention the use of poppy seeds
as a remedy for flatulence (Leake, 1952, p. 72) and the application
of a mixture of opium pods and fly excreta as a sedative for children
(Wright, 1968, p. 65). That the effects of the plant were known to the
ancients is further supported by the legend of Demeter, the goddess
of agriculture and fertility, who, while searching for her daughter
Persephone, forgot her sorrow after tasting bitter gum oozing from the
poppy (Levinthal, 1985, p. 562). One of the clearest and earliest
accounts of the poppy can be found in *The Greek Herbal of Dioscorides*.
Written by a Greek physician in the Roman legions of the Emperor
Nero during the 1st century A.D., this remarkable work outlined

hundreds of remedies derived from plant, animal, and mineral sources, serving as an authoritative reference for physicians for over 1500 years. Dioscorides described some of the effects of Mekon Agrios and Emeros, the opium poppy, as follows:

> Ye seed of the black Poppy beaten small is given to drink with wine for ye flux of ye belly, & ye womanish flux. It is applied unto such as cannot sleep with water upon ye forehead & the temples, but the liquor itself is more cooling & thickening & drying. A little of it taken as much as a grain of Ervum, is a pain-easer & a sleep causer, & a digester, helping coughes, & Coeliacall affections. But being drunk too much, it hurts, making men lethargicall & it kills. It is helpful also for ye headaches. . . . But being put up with ye finger for a suppository, it causeth sleep [c. 77 A.D., p. 458].

Thus, the benefits as well as some of the possible harmful results of opium administration were recognized.

During the centuries that followed, the use of opium spread throughout the world. Avicenna, the great Arabian physician of the middle ages, noted that "The most powerful of the stupefacients is opium" (n.d., p. 527). In sixteenth-century Europe, the well-known Paracelsus popularized a drink containing opium, wine, and spices as treatment for a variety of diseases, calling the mixture laudanum —"something to be praised" (Levinthal, 1985, p. 563).

Thomas Sydenham (1624–1689) expressed almost a religious enthusiasm for opium in his *Medical Observations Concerning the History and the Cure of Acute Disease,* stating:

> And here I cannot but break out in praise of the great God, the Giver of all good things, who hath granted to the human race, as a comfort in their afflictions, no medicine of the value of opium, either in regard to the number of diseases that it can control, or its efficiency in extirpating them. . . . So necessary an instrument is opium in the hands of a skilful man, that medicine would be a cripple without it; and whoever understands it well, will do more with it alone than he could well hope to do from any single medicine [1676, p. 173].

Although the potential harmful effects of opium were recognized, little was done about controlling its use before the twentieth century. Laudanum-based medications were popular and readily obtainable from apothecaries in the guise of patent remedies, with attractive names such as Godfrey's Cordial, Mrs. Winslow's Soothing Syrup, a Pennysworth of Peace, Mother Bailey's Quieting Syrup, Dalby's Carminative, and McMunn's Elixer of Opium (Hayter, 1968; Levinthal,

1985). One of the most notorious of these opium compounds, Dover's Powder, was concocted by the pirate-physician Thomas Dover (c. 1660–1742), whose life of adventure has been associated with the original story of Robinson Crusoe (Osler, 1896). First recommended as a treatment for gout over 250 years ago, this famous remedy has a picturesque formula, which reads as follows:

> Take Opium one Ounce, Salt-Petre and Tartar vitriolated, each four Ounces, Ipocacuana one Ounce, Liquorish one Ounce. Put the Salt-Petre and Tartar into a red-hot Mortar, stirring them with a Spoon till they have done flaming.—Then powder them very fine; after that slice in your Opium; grind these to a Powder, and then mix the other Powders with these. Dose from forty to sixty or seventy Grains in a glass of White-Wine Posset, going to Bed.—Covering up warm, and drinking a Quart or three Pints of the Posset-Drink while sweating [Dover, 1733, p. 14].

Dover's Powder continued to be cited in the twentieth century, prescribed as "pulvis ipecacuanhoe et opii" for the relief of pain (Clendening, 1935, p. 69) and for its benefits as an expectorant (p. 164).

During the nineteenth century, easy accessibility to opium-containing compounds resulted in their frequent misuse to sedate infants and children and in the development of widespread opium dependence throughout all strata of European society (Levinthal, 1985). Indeed, such was the cavalier attitude toward the drug that Berridge was prompted to comment that "Opium was the aspirin of the time" (Berridge, 1982, p. 2). During this period, many writers came to believe that opium could aid the creative process (overtones of LSD and the 1960s), a notion that was reinforced by Thomas De Quincey, in his famous *Confessions of an English Opium-Eater* (1821). Hayter, commenting on De Quincey, wrote:

> De Quincey was the first writer, and he is perhaps still the only one, to study deliberately, from within his personal experience, the way in which dreams and visions are formed, how opium helps to form them and intensifies them, and how they are then re-composed and used in conscious art. . . .
> It was his belief that opium dreams and rêveries could be in themselves a creative process both analogous to, and leading to, literary creation. . . .
> De Quincey became the prophet of opium [1968, pp. 103–104].

The manner in which opium ingestion and addiction may have influenced the imagination, originality, productivity, and lives of Samuel Taylor Coleridge, John Keats, George Crabbe, Edgar Allan Poe, and other literary greats of this era has been discussed by Hayter in the book *Opium and the Romantic Imagination*, whose concluding words included the declaration that "Their paradises may have been wholly or partly artificial; their hells were real" (1968, p. 342).

The shameful and degrading history of the Opium Trade Wars between England and China during the mid-nineteenth century, briefly discussed by Levinthal (1985), is a sad commentary on human weaknesses and human greed. The medical benefits of opium, on the other hand, are not to be overlooked. William Heberden, author of the well-known *Commentaries on the History and Cure of Diseases*, in which is contained his famous and unequaled description of angina pectoris, stated that "Opium taken at bed-time will prevent the attacks [of angina] at night" (1802, p. 369). Elsewhere, in a previously unpublished essay found amongst his manuscripts, Heberden also wrote the following:

> Opium is far from being the least of those blessings with which Providence has furnished us for the mitigation of the various sufferings, to which the human form is liable. There are specifics, or certain cures for few of our ails, but opium affords some relief to all [Paulshock, 1983, p. 55].

Similar praise has been expressed during the present century by Logan Clendening, who commented that "Few physicians would be sufficiently hard-hearted to practice medicine without opium" (1935, p. 69).

In the early years of the nineteenth century, preliminary accounts describing the isolation of a salt-forming base from opium were reported by Friedrich Wilhelm Adam Sertürner, a German pharmacist. Several years later, Sertürner (1817) published an important article entitled "On morphium, a salt-like base, and meconic acid as chief constituents of opium" in which he gave the details of his method for isolating the alkaloid within opium that was responsible for its narcotic, analgesic, and toxic properties. Naming this substance *Morphium* after Morpheus, the God of Sleep and Dreams, Sertürner laid the foundation for alkaloidal chemistry with his landmark discovery (Hanzlik, 1929; Lockemann, 1951). In order to achieve uniform nomenclature, Gay-Lussac, the eminent French chemist, shortly thereafter proposed that as more plant bases were identified, their names should end in the suffix "ine," thus resulting in "morphium" being renamed "morphine" (Sneader, 1985, p. 7).

Morphine, the standard to which other analgesics are compared, is active in relieving pain when administered by mouth, by rectum, and by the intravenous, intramuscular and spinal routes. The availability of hypodermic syringes in the mid-nineteenth century (see "Syringes and Hypodermic Injections" in this volume) provided a precise and effective way of dispensing the drug. The benefits of morphine, however, were accompanied by troublesome medical and psychological problems resulting from the drug and from drug addiction. Indeed, as David Courtwright put it, "A syringe of morphine was, in a very real sense, a magic wand. Though it could cure little, it could relieve anything; doctors and patients alike were tempted to overuse" (1982, p. 47).

An extensive historical and literature review of scientific studies devoted to opiates over the last two centuries, with particular attention to the problems of opiate addiction, was outlined by Kramer (1980). In addition, therapeutic applications of morphine are continually being re-examined, addressing issues related to the control of pain in cancer patients, the management of intractable pain, the pharmacodynamic effects and dosing schedules of newer morphine preparations, and the most suitable route of drug administration for a specific type of pain (Wilkes and Levy, 1984).

Writers and poets have frequently invoked the mystery and aura associated with the poppy and its derivatives to convey the images they wish to portray. In Shakespeare's *Othello*, Iago says,

> Not poppy, nor mandragora,
> Nor all the drowsy syrups of the world,
> Shall ever medicine thee to that sweet sleep
> Which thou ow'dst yesterday.
>
> Act III, Scene iii, Line 331

John Keats, in his poem *To Sleep*, wrote:

> O soothest Sleep! if so it please thee,
>   close,
> In midst of this thine hymn, my willing
>   eyes,
> Or wait the amen, ere thy poppy throws
>   Around my bed its dewy charities.
>
> [1819, p. 142]

More recently, Sylvia Plath, in a poem entitled *The Surgeon at*

2 A.M., wrote that "The angels of morphia have borne him up" (1961, p. 171).

Peter Mere Latham once wrote, although in a somewhat different context, that "poisons and medicines are oftentimes the same substances given with different intents" (1861, p. 324). Such a view might be applied to opium and morphine preparations which, when administered for the relief of pain, serve as effective and beneficial medications, but when given to perpetuate an unfortunate medically induced addiction or an illicit drug habit may result in enormous medical and psychological hardships. Thus, this same group of agents when "given with different intents" may serve as either a medicine or a poison—a blessing or a curse.

9

Iron: The Legendary Metal

> Then give them great meals of beef and iron and
> steel, they will eat like wolves and fight like devils.
> [Shakespeare—*Henry* V, Act III,
> Scene vii, Line 166.]

A NCIENT legends ascribed extraordinary therapeutic powers to iron. In one such story, Christian recounts how Melampus, a shepherd supposed to have supernatural power, was directed by a vulture to scrape the rust off a knife, dissolve it in wine, and administer it to Iphyclus so he "would be lusty and capable of begetting children" (1903, pp. 176–177). Aside from such mythologic references, manuscripts from early times contain prescriptions in which iron was dispensed for a variety of ailments. The Ebers Papyrus of ancient Egypt listed iron as an ingredient for the relief of baldness (Fairbanks, Fahey, and Beutler, 1971, p. 2). An Assyrian medical text, according to Krause, recommended the following remedy for the treatment of photophobia, an abnormal sensitivity of the eye to light: "powdered iron ore, iron sulphate, copper, lead, arsenic, tamarisk-seed, laurel-seed, in the suet of the kidney of a black ox" (1934, p. 51).

Hippocrates was said to have used iron medicinally as a styptic, a substance that controls bleeding, with a similar application described by Pliny the Elder during the first century A.D. (Fairbanks et al., 1971, pp. 4–5). Indeed, this use of iron was still discussed nearly two thousand

73

years later in a pharmacology textbook of the late nineteenth century. According to that work a preparation of subsulphate of iron known as Monsel's solution, applied externally, "is one of the most efficacious styptics we can employ" (Biddle, 1880, pp. 152–153). Other medical conditions for which iron was used during the period of the Roman Empire included skin disorders, diarrheas, fevers, wounds, and infections of various types. Several hundred years later, the famous *Canon of Medicine* by the Arabian physician Avicenna stated that "ferruginous waters impart strength to the internal organs, prevent stomach trouble, and stimulate the appetite. They resolve the spleen and are beneficial for those who cannot cohabit properly" (n.d., p. 227).

Legends and superstitions gave rise to the notion that Mars, the god of war, had imbued iron with force and strength, with the result that medications known as saffron of mars, tincture of the syrup of mars with tartar, and crocus martis were administered in the hope that they would impart these attributes to patients who had symptoms of weakness and loss of vigor (Christian, 1903; Haden, 1938). An early eighteenth-century reference to one of these remedies describes it as follows: "Crocus martis is prepared in either of the following three ways: by exposing plates of iron to dew; by sprinkling iron filings with rain water or water and honey; by heating iron white hot and plunging into melted sulphur. This last form is red and on this account thought a better medicine" (Christian, 1903, p. 179).

The use of iron to treat patients with anemia is closely associated with a disease called chlorosis, a form of anemia primarily effecting young girls, one of the earliest descriptions of which was written in the sixteenth century by Johannes Lange (1485–1565). Referring to this disorder as "De Morbo Virgineo" (1554, p. 445), an affliction "perculiar to virgins" (p. 446), Lange described the face of a girl with this disease

> as if exsanguinated, sadly paled, the heart trembles with every movement of her body, and the arteries of her temples pulsate, & she is seized with dyspnoea in dancing or climbing the stairs, her stomach loathes food and particularly meat, & the legs, especially at the ankles, become edematous at night [1554, pp. 445–446].

According to Fowler, the name chlorosis, which comes from the Greek word for green, was given to this disorder by Jean Vavandal in 1620 (1936, p. 170), for which reason it has often been referred to as the green-sickness. Whether it was because of the previously discussed association of the Greek god Mars with iron, or whether it was due to the observed similarity of the color of blood and bloodstains to the color of iron (Fairbanks et. al., 1971, p. 5), the empiric observation that iron could be used as a remedy for chlorosis preceded by many years any understanding of iron metabolism and hemoglobin synthesis. The English physician Thomas Sydenham is generally credited with so introducing iron for the treatment of anemia, specifically for chlorosis:

> I comfort the blood and the spirits belonging to it by giving a chalybeate [i.e., something containing or charged with iron] thirty days running. This is sure to do good. To the worn-out and languid blood it gives a spur or fillip, whereby the animal spirits, which before lay prostrate and sunken under their own weight, are raised and excited. Clear proof of this is found in the effects of steel upon chlorosis. The pulse gains strength and frequency, the surface warmth, the face (no longer pale and deathlike) a fresh ruddy colour. . . .
>
> Next to steel in substance, I prefer a syrup. This is made by steeping iron or steel filings in cold Rhenish wine. When the wine is sufficiently impregnated, strain the liquor; add sugar; and boil to the consistency of a syrup [1682, pp. 97–98].

Present use of the phrase "tired blood" may well be a direct descendant of this picturesque description written over 300 years ago.

Early contributions to understanding iron metabolism were made in the first half of the eighteenth century by Lemery and Geoffry, who demonstrated that iron was present in the ash of blood, and by Menghini, who showed that the amount of iron in the blood of experimental animals could be increased by feeding them iron-containing foods (Christian, 1903, pp. 178–179). Such observations supported the use of iron therapy as recommended earlier by Sydenham.

During the 1830s, still many years before quantitative tests to determine red blood cell count and hemoglobin level were available for clinical use, the Frenchman Pierre Blaud described the nature of the blood in chlorosis and the principles of iron therapy for treating this disease:

> But in all these cases it comes from a vicious sanguinification, the result of which is an imperfect fluid, where the serosity predominates, where the coloring principle is lacking and which is no longer suited to excite suitably the organism and carry on the regular exercise of its functions. The treatment is ferruginous preparations, modifiers of the organism, which give back to the blood the exciting principle which it has lost, that is to say the coloring substance. When

one knows the importance of the blood and the rôle which it plays in the organic scene of life, when one knows that this fluid is the exciting agent of all our parts, and the prime mover of all their functions, one is little astonished at the trouble manifested when the conditions necessary to its influence no longer exist in its composition and that it lacks some one of the elements. Here the coloring matter is lacking. It is a clinical fact, which we know to be beyond doubt and from here arise all the functional disorders [Christian, 1903, pp. 179–180].

Thirty patients were cured in ten to thirty-two days after receiving Blaud's new formulation, a remedy which called for equal parts of iron sulphate and potassium carbonate pulverized to a fine powder to which mucilage tragacanth was added, with the resulting mixture divided into pills each containing "the equivalent of 5 grains (0.3 Gm.) of ferrous sulphate, or approximately 2 grains (0.1 Gm.) of ferrous carbonate" (Haden, 1938, p. 1060). This prescription has been little improved upon in the intervening years.

Testimony to the success of Blaud's preparation can be found in the American edition of a famous German textbook of medicine by Dr. Felix von Niemeyer: "For more than twenty years I have used *Blaud's* pills almost exclusively in chlorosis, and have witnessed such brilliant results from them in a large number of cases, that I have never found any opportunity to experiment with other articles" (1881, p. 808). Blaud's pills and chlorosis were also well known enough to be referred to in Somerset Maugham's novel *Of Human Bondage*: "I say, you are anaemic . . . I'll have to dose you with Blaud's Pills" (1915, p. 415), with later reference to "that green skin of yours" (p. 417).

The field of hematology was probably launched in 1674 with Antonj van Leeuwenhoek's visualization and description of red blood cells under the microscope (Garrison, 1929, p. 254). During the latter half of the nineteenth century, Funke discovered the nature of hemoglobin, Hoppe-Seyler obtained hemoglobin in crystalline form, William Gowers invented the hemoglobinometer, and Georges Hayem described the morphology of red blood cells in anemia, all important contributions toward a more rational understanding of iron metabolism (Fowler, 1936, p. 171). A most significant microscopic description of the blood of patients with chlorosis was given in 1867 by Johann Duncan of St. Petersburg. As quoted by Fairbanks et al., Duncan asserted "that in chlorosis every single blood cell contains less pigment than is in the blood corpuscles of healthy individuals" (1971, p. 18). At the close of the nineteenth century, a little-known work by Ralph Stockman at the School of Medicine in Edinburgh demonstrated that the hemoglobin level could be increased in women with chlorosis by giving them iron therapy (Stockman, 1893). Indeed, Meulengracht in Copenhagen was so convinced of the specificity of iron therapy in patients with this disorder that he wrote: "On the whole the effect of iron treatment is relatively so certain in chlorosis that if it is absent we may suspect that some other agency is at work simultaneously or we may doubt whether it is really a case of true chlorosis" (1923, p. 609).

Several years later, Heath, Strauss, and Castle at the Thorndike Memorial Laboratory and Harvard Medical School attempted

first, to describe the dosage of iron which may be given parenterally in hypochromic anemia, and to compare it with the dosage by mouth; secondly, to determine the fate of iron administered parenterally, and establish a quantitative basis for the better knowledge of this type of deficiency [1932, p. 1293].

These investigators presented evidence that "iron given therapeutically in hypochromic anemia is supplying a deficiency, and is thus being made available for the normal manufacture of necessary hemoglobin molecules" (1932, p. 1308), later noting that the "relationship of the deficient substance, iron, to the deficiency itself, which is mainly in the circulating hemoglobin, can be expressed in a quantitative fashion" (1932, p. 1310). Thus, it was convincingly established that absorbed iron in patients with iron deficiency anemia was quantitatively utilized in the synthesis of hemoglobin.

The diagnosis of chlorosis is rarely if ever made at present. Whether improved diagnostic procedures in patients with iron deficiency anemias now permit other and more precise etiologic diagnoses to be made in place of this disorder, or whether dietary or cultural changes in recent years have reduced the frequency with which this disease actually occurs, may never be known with certainty (Fowler, 1936; Fairbanks et al., 1971). However, regardless of the reason, this now all-but-vanished ailment has served a valuable purpose—through it, much of present-day understanding and use of iron therapy and metabolism have evolved.

The principal application of iron in current medical practice is for the therapy of patients with iron-deficiency anemias. Most of the

information necessary for the treatment of such patients was well established by the middle of the twentieth century, although the use of
radioactive isotopes of iron since that time has extended our knowledge
of iron metabolism still further. Truly, with its long and interesting
history and with all the benefits it has bestowed, there is perhaps some
merit in the appellation given to iron as "the metal of heaven" (Fairbanks et al., 1971, p. 2).

10

Colchicine and Gout

A perverse, ungrateful, maleficent malady
[George H. Ellwanger, 1897]

HIPPOCRATES (460–370 B.C.) has been credited with the first description of gout in man, although previously "podagra," as gout was then called, had been known as a disease involving the joints of animals (Schnitker, 1936, p. 90). The word "podagra" is formed from a picturesque combination of the Greek word "pous" (pod), foot, and "agra," seizure, meaning therefore a foot seizure, the classic, well known form of the disease.

For over 2,000 years, religious, magic, and empiric cures for gout abounded. These included manipulation, acupuncture, cautery, electricity, blood-letting, and the application of materials such as horseradish, mustard powders, and animal dung (Rodnan and Benedek, 1963, p. 327). An unusual treatment was described in an early eighteenth-century textbook by Richard Bradley: "*Columba*, or the Pigeon or Dove, is seldom recommended by any Physician; but to apply it warm and Bleeding to the Bottoms of the Feet to such Persons as are troubled with the Gout, Vertigo, and Palsie, where it proves of good Use" (1730, p. 157). During the early nineteenth century, leeches were applied to the knee of the afflicted patient. The benefits of soaking a gouty limb in cold water was noted by others (Pfeiffer, 1985, pp. 48, 175).

It was not until the thirteenth century that the term "gout" was actually introduced, originating from the Latin *gutta* meaning "drop." This may have been a reference to the then-popular belief that drops of "bad humors" from the body are deposited in the afflicted part during a gouty attack (Schnitker, 1936, p. 91). In discussing the cause of gout, the great Thomas Sydenham wrote in his classic publication A *Treatise on Gout and Dropsy*:

> Gouty patients are, generally, either old men, or men who have so worn themselves out in youth as to have brought on a premature old age—of such dissolute habits none being more common that the premature and excessive indulgence in venery, and the like exhausting passions. Add to this the inter-mission or the sudden abandonment of those exercises to which from their youth upwards they had been accustomed. Whilst these were kept up the blood was invigorated, and the tone of the body rendered firm and steady. When however they were dropped, the animal spirits gave way, the frame lost tone, and the assimilation became imperfect. . . .
>   Add to this that great eaters are liable to gout; and, of these, the costive [constipated, slow] more especially. Eating as they used to eat when in full exercise, their digestion is naturally impaired. Even in these cases simple glut-tony, and the free use of food, although common incentives, by no means so frequently pave the way for gout as reckless and inordinate drinking [1683, pp. 129–130].

Other references about gout cited by Rodnan and Benedek exhibit similar themes, with the disease looked upon as "the legitimate off-spring of luxury and intemperance" and as the consequence of "the dissolute and voluptuous Indulgence of sensual Appetites" (1963, p. 318).

Clarification of an important relationship between gout and the amount of uric acid in the body was documented during the nineteenth century by the London physician Alfred Baring Garrod, writing in his masterful book entitled A *Treatise on Gout and Rheumatic Gout* that "*the blood in gout is invariably rich in uric acid*" (1876, p. 91). Meas-uring the level of uric acid in blood has remained to this day an important test in clinical practice for confirming the diagnosis of gout.

The history of colchicine therapy almost parallels the 2,000–2,500 year history of gout. Colchicine, an effective drug still used in the management of gout, is obtained from the plant *Colchicum autum-nale*, so named because it grew in Colchis, a region on the eastern shore of the Black Sea celebrated in Greek mythology. Early accounts of this plant are at times confusing, owing "to the existence of several terms for botanicals which may or may not have been identical to *C. autumnale*, eg. hermodactyl, surinjan and ephemeron [ephemerum]" (Rodnan and Benedek, 1970, p. 145). According to Hartung (1954), Nicander of the second century B.C. described this plant in his *Alexipharmaca*, a work on plant poisons, and *The Greek Herbal of Dioscorides* mentions "Colchicum, which some call Ephemerum" (Dioscorides, *c.* 77 A.D., p. 481). The Byzantine physician Alexander of Tralles of the sixth century A.D. is credited with being one of the first, if not the first, to use this plant in treating certain forms of arthritis (Hartung, 1954). Alexander prescribed hermodactyl—Hermes after the god Mercury, and dactylus, meaning "a finger"—administering it in a manner very similar to that in which present-day colchicine is used. Evidence was cited by Schnitker (1936, pp. 101–102) and Hartung (1954, pp. 193–194) indicating that *Colchicum autumnale* and hermodactyl were actually one and the same plant, thus providing support for the supposition that colchicine was used nearly 1,500 years ago in the management of joint disorders. Although hermodactyl was effective, it severely irritated the stomach and intestines and thus had limited application.

The reintroduction of colchicum as a modern therapeutic agent occurred in the eighteenth century with the publication of Anton von Stoerck's book entitled *An Essay on the Use and Effects of the Root of the Colchicum Autumnale, or Meadow-Saffron* (1764), with the drug initially being cited for its diuretic action rather than for its effect in gout. Shortly thereafter, a French military officer named Nicholas Husson (or d'Husson) concocted a secret remedy called "Eau médicinale" that was used not only for treating gout but also for a variety of unrelated disorders (1783). During this period, other similar preparations were known by names such as Portland powder, Wilson's tincture, Reynold's specific, and Laville's tincture (Schnitker, 1936).

In the early nineteenth century, Mr. John Want, Surgeon to the Northern Dispensary of London, demonstrated that the effective ingredient in "Eau médicinale" was colchicum and that "experiments have already been made [with the plant] in at least *forty cases*, followed by results of the most satisfactory nature, the paroxysms being always removed" (1815, p. 89–90). Thereafter, the latter replaced previously described nostrums for treating gouty attacks, receiving the endorsement of many, including royalty. Sir Astley Cooper, attending the future King George IV of England in the early nineteenth century, related the following story:

> He [George IV] was a good judge of the medicine which would best suit him. . . .
> He suffered much from rheumatism and gout, but the colchicum relieved him.
> One morning, when he had rheumatism in his hip, and there was a doubt about the propriety of giving colchicum, he said, 'Gentlemen, I have borne your half-measures long enough to please you—now I will please myself, and take colchicum,' which he did, and was soon relieved [Cooper, 1843, pp. 351–352].

The legitimacy of the claim that Benjamin Franklin, a sufferer from gout himself, was responsible for introducing colchicum in some form into the United States is problematical, although he was in Europe during the period that this form of treatment was being used (Wallace, 1968).

In 1820, Pellétier and Caventou isolated the active ingredient from colchicum. Thirteen years later, Geiger identified this substance as an alkaloid and proposed naming it *colchicine* (Rodnan and Benedek, 1970, p. 152).

An observation made by Garrod over one hundred years ago is still pertinent. Commenting upon the therapeutic specificity of this drug and its ability to assist in making a differential diagnosis, he wrote: "I would even go the length of asserting that we may sometimes diagnose gouty inflammation from any other form by noting the influence of colchicum upon its progress" (1876, p. 321).

Colchicine is also an antimitotic agent and has been used experimentally to study normal and abnormal cell division. However, it is its unique and still incompletely understood anti-inflammatory effects during acute attacks of gout and its ability to serve as a prophylactic agent against such attacks that have enabled the drug to survive for nearly 1,500 years as part of the physician's therapeutic armamentarium.

11

Atropine, Witches, and Mystical Plants

THERAPEUTICALLY active and potentially toxic belladonna alkaloids—principally atropine, hyoscyamine, and scopolamine—are
found within many plants of the nightshade family. The better known
of these plants—*Datura stramonium* (Jimson weed), *Hyoscyamus niger*
(black henbane), *Atropa belladonna* (deadly nightshade), and the legendary and now medically obsolete *Mandragora officinarum* (mandrake)—have fascinating and colorful histories that extend as far back
as ancient Egyptian and Grecian times. As a result of their narcotic,
hypnotic, and hallucinogenic properties, these plants have not only
found medical uses but have also been linked to various magical and
religious beliefs and myths, acquiring an extraordinary reputation.

Numerous tales and superstitions have been associated with the
plant known as mandragora or mandrake, made famous particularly
by those delving in magic and witchcraft. Superstitions about mandrake
were in part an example of the doctrine or law of signatures, in which
plants that suggested by their color or shape certain parts of the body
were used to treat the organ they resembled. Since the roots of the
mandrake were thought to look like a human figure, the belief arose
that this plant could exercise supernatural powers over the human
mind and body (Schultes and Hofmann, 1979). It was also believed
that those removing the plant from the ground would die, for which
reason this task had to be done by a dog. In addition (Figure 11.1),
to avoid hearing the piercing cry of the mandrake as it was pulled from
the earth and to avoid being knocked down by the smell that accompanied the cry, those standing in the vicinity were instructed to stuff
their ears and to position themselves windward (Heiser, 1969, p. 134).

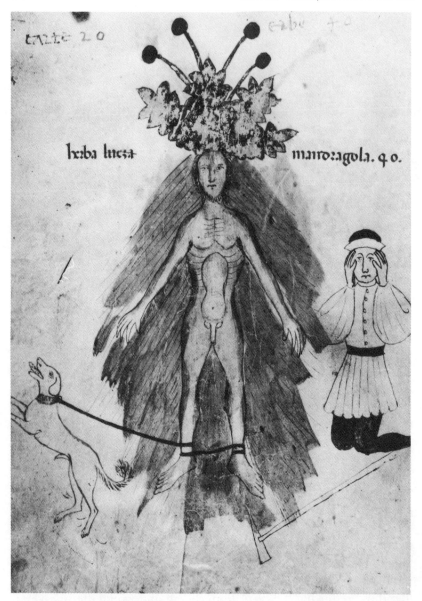

FIG. 11.1. The legend of the mandrake was portrayed in a fourteenth-century manuscript, showing a dog tied to the root of a mandrake plant and a man covering his ears to avoid hearing the cry of the plant as it was pulled from the earth. *Source:* Aldini Manuscript 211, c. 20v. Courtesy of Biblioteca Universitaria, Pavia, Italy.

Dioscorides, nearly two thousand years ago, included a description of the narcotic properties of the mandrake in his discussion of the plant: "Using a Cyathus [a small, long-handled cup or ladle] of it for such as cannot sleep, or are grievously pained, & upon whom being cut, or cauterized they wish to make a non-feeling pain" (*c*. 77 A.D., p. 473). He also referred to the sexual powers of the mandrake, noting that "the root [of the plant] seems to be a maker of love medicines" (p. 473). Indeed, according to Heiser, "one of the most important properties attached to the plant was the power of influencing sexual relations—either as an aphrodisiac, a cure for sterility, or a philtre for gaining the favor of one's beloved" (1969, p. 133). This attribute of the plant was similarly suggested in the Bible, in *The Song of Solomon*, 7:13:

> The mandrakes give forth fragrance,
>   and over our doors are all choice fruits,
> new as well as old,
>   which I have laid up for you, O my beloved.

The root of the mandrake contains hyoscyamine, scopolamine, and another alkaloid called mandragorine (Tyler, Brady, and Robbers, 1981, p. 209). Although reportedly still used in parts of southern Europe and in China (Heiser, 1969, pp. 135–136), the mandrake has not had a place in pharmaceutics for many years. It still, however, has a secure foothold in legend and literature, and long after many of today's remedies have disappeared from memory, such verses as these from Shakespeare's plays will continue to remind us of this unusual plant:

> Give me to drink mandragora. . . .
> That I might sleep out this great gap of time
> My Antony is away.
>   [*Antony and Cleopatra*, Act I, Scene v, Line 4]
>
> And shrieks like mandrakes' torn out of the earth,
> That living mortals, hearing them, run mad.
>   *Romeo and Juliet*, Act IV, Scene iii, Line 47]

Hyoscyamus niger, known commonly as black henbane although also referred to as stinking nightshade, stinking Roger, and fetid nightshade, was mentioned by Dioscorides (*c*. 77 A.D., pp. 464–465) for treating a variety of painful ailments, for which purposes it remained popular until the late Middle Ages. During the latter period, the plant was used as an ingredient in an anesthetic agent, and up to three to four hundred years ago reference was still made to its effect in easing the pain of toothache (Heiser, 1969, p. 150). However, as Schultes and Hofmann noted, "Its best-known use was as one of the main ingredients permitting the witches of medieval times to experience hallucinations and other effects of intoxication" (1979, p. 87). In the first century A.D., the potency and toxicity of the plant were attested to by Pliny, as quoted by Heiser: "For my own part, I hold it to be dangerous medicine, and not to be used but with great heed and discretion. For this is certainly knowne, that, if one takes in drinke more than four leaves, thereof, it will put him beside himself" (Heiser, 1969, p. 149).

The active principles of henbane have been shown to be hyoscyamine and to a lesser extent scopolamine (Tyler, Brady, and Robbers, 1981, p. 207). Late nineteenth-century pharmacology texts (Biddle, 1880, pp. 74–76; Bartholow, 1882, pp. 360–363) mention that it contains no special advantages over other related plants, and in addition, is difficult to procure and expensive.

Of the various species of Datura, probably the best known in medicine is *Datura stramonium*, the Jamestown or Jimson weed, which contains hyoscyamine, scopolamine, and small amounts of atropine. Called stinkweed by some because of its evil odor, this plant was also described by Dioscorides in his much-quoted source book of medical botany: "The root being drank with wine ye quantity of a dragm, hath ye power to effect not unpleasant fantasies. But 2 dragms being drank, make one beside himself for three days & 4 being drank kill him" (c. 77 A.D., p. 470).

The narcotic and hallucinogenic effects of *Datura* were subsequently recognized and reported on many occasions over the years. Schultes and Hofmann cite a sixteenth-century quotation in which Acosta described unique actions of the plant upon the brain and nervous system, stating that "he who partakes of it is deprived of his reason for a long time, laughing or weeping or sleeping . . . at times he appears to be in his right mind, but really being out of it" (1980, p. 283).

Perhaps one of the most unusual accounts of the hallucinogenic effects produced by this plant appeared in *The History and Present State of Virginia* by Robert Beverley. The plant—the Jamestown or

Jimson weed—was mistakenly gathered for a salad by a group of soldiers with the following bizarre results:

> [A]nd some of them eat plentifully of it, the Effect of which was a very pleasant Comedy; for they turn'd natural Fools upon it for several Days: One would blow up a Feather in the Air; another wou'd dart Straws at it with much Fury; and another stark naked was sitting up in a Corner, like a Monkey, grinning and making Mows at them; a Fourth would fondly kiss, and paw his Companions, and snear in their Faces, with a Countenance more antick, than any in a *Dutch* Droll. In this frantick Condition they were confined, lest they should in their Folly destroy themselves; though it was observed, that all their Actions were full of Innocence and good Nature. Indeed, they were not very cleanly; for they would have wallow'd in their own Excrements, if they had not been prevented. A Thousand such simple Tricks they play'd, and after Eleven Days, return'd to themselves again, not remembring any thing that had pass'd [Beverley, 1705, p. 24].

In more recent years, patients with signs and symptoms of atropine poisoning following ingestion of Jimson weed have been described as "hot as a hare, blind as a bat, dry as a bone, red as a beet and mad as a wet hen" (Arena, 1963, p. 183), referring to the high temperatures that may be detected in children, the eye symptoms, the dryness of the mucous membranes, the flushing of the skin and occasional rash, and the psychotic behavior.

The extensive role of several species of Datura in medicine and religious rites in the New World has been reviewed by Schultes and Hofmann. In the American Southwest, the Zuni Indian tribe referred to *Datura inoxia* as *a-neg-la-kya* and prized it as an anesthetic, as a poultice for wounds and bruises, and as a hallucinogen. Similarly, a number of Indian tribes in the Southwest and in Mexico use these plants to induce visions and intoxication during adolescent initiation rites and during ceremonial functions (1980, pp. 285–286).

Not too many years ago, those seeking additional ways to obtain hallucinogenic and psychedelic experiences discovered *Asthmador*, an old-fashioned remedy for the treatment of asthma. This stramonium–belladonna mixture, dispensed in the form of a powder that could be smoked or burned so as to permit its vapors to be inhaled, contained the active principles scopolamine and atropine. As news spread of the availability of the substance without a prescription, cases of poisoning and intoxication of teen-agers who ingested it were reported. Symptoms ranged from a "high" to a dangerous psychotic reaction requiring hospitalization (Koff, 1966; Goldsmith, Frank, and Ungerleider, 1968;

Cummins, Obetz, and Wilson, 1968). In 1968, the seriousness of this problem prompted the United States Food and Drug Administration to remove such asthma powders from their status as over-the-counter medications and to place them in the prescription-drug category (Tyler, Brady, and Robbers, 1981, p. 209).

In the sixteenth century, John Gerarde (or Gerard), writing in *The Herball or Generall Historie of Plantes*, described the effects of the plant known today as *Atropa belladonna*, well-known as a source of atropine and other belladonna alkaloids: "This kinde of Nightshade causeth sleepe, troubleth the minde, bringeth madnes[s] if a fewe of the berries be inwardly taken, but if mo be giuen they also kill and bring present death" (1597, p. 270). Gerarde mentioned several different names by which this plant was called—sleeping Nightshade, deadly or raging Nightshade, Dwale, and Bella dona.

The origin of the name *Atropa belladonna* has always aroused interest. Because of the poisonous attributes of the plant, Linné named it *Atropa* after Atropos, one of the three fates in Greek mythology, who "cut the thread of life when a man's course was run" (Forbes, 1977, p. 403). The most frequent explanation given for the term *belladonna*, the Italian for beautiful lady, relates the name to the practice of Italian ladies of putting belladonna juice in their eyes in order to dilate the pupils and make themselves more alluring or beautiful. Forbes (1977), however, also mentions other possible origins for the epithet—that the juices or distilled extract of the plant may have been used as a cosmetic by the ladies of Venice, that the poisonous qualities of the plant were exploited by a famous poisoner in Italy to destroy beautiful women, and that beautiful women who took an extract of the plant developed sexual fantasies.

During the first half of the nineteenth century, atropine was isolated from the roots of belladonna by Mein, a German apothecary (Sneader, 1985, p. 120). As additional belladonna alkaloids were identified, an extensive body of literature was accumulated on the pharmacologic actions of these substances, known today as muscarinic agents because they inhibit the muscarinic actions of acetylcholine. At various times, they have also been called *anticholinergic*, *antispasmodic*, *parasympatholytic*, or *antiparasympathetic* agents, names that in part describe their actions. The best known of these drugs is atropine, for which reason the term *atropine-like* has sometimes been applied to all the members of this group.

The belladonna alkaloids have been prescribed in a wide variety of clinical conditions. Their lack of selectivity, however, has meant that undesirable side effects frequently accompany the benefits that are obtained, thus limiting their use. In treating diseases of the central nervous system, the belladonna alkaloids have been helpful in the management of Parkinson's disease, although levodopa is currently a preferred therapy for this disorder. Scopolamine has been an effective prophylactic for motion sickness, used in recent years in the form of a skin patch. As preoperative medications, the belladonna agents have been useful in preventing excessive salivation and in reducing secretions of the respiratory tract while patients are receiving anesthesia. These drugs have also been administered as an ingredient in various "cold" remedies for symptomatic relief from secretions and congestion of the respiratory passages. Eye drops containing an antimuscarinic agent produce mydriasis (dilatation of the pupil) and cyclopegia (paralysis of the ciliary muscles), effects that have both diagnostic and therapeutic applications; as mentioned, such uses might be traced to those that gave rise to the name belladonna. The administration of these agents to reduce the secretion of gastric acid in patients with peptic ulcer disease has now largely been replaced by the use of H_2-receptor antagonists. However, a large number of proprietary and over-the-counter remedies still contain belladonna alkaloids since they relieve the painful and uncomfortable symptoms associated with "spasm" or increased tone of smooth muscles in the organs of the gastrointestinal and genitourinary tracts.

The action of atropine upon the heart has found a use in the treatment of patients with slow heart rates. Von Bezold and Bloebaum in 1867 and Schmiedeberg in 1870, as noted in references cited by Klein, Barret, Ryan, and Flessas (1975, p. 200), demonstrated that the cardiac effects of vagal stimulation are blocked by atropine, although interestingly enough, prior to the acceleration of the heart rate, a transient period of slowing may first occur. This phenomenon was described by Bartholow a few years later in his book A *Practical Treatise on Materia Medica and Therapeutics*:

> It [atropia] affects the circulation in a remarkable manner. In some subjects a decided slowing of the heart takes place immediately after the administration of a considerable dose (atropia hypodermically), and in all, most probably, an instantaneous retardation of the pulse-rate, but a very decided rise in the number of pulsations quickly follows [1882, p. 349].

McGuigan (1921) indicated that small doses of atropine slow the heart by an action on the vagus center in the medulla of the brain. Additional studies of the biphasic response to atropine demonstrated that the rate decreased when a small dose of atropine was given or the drug was administered slowly, an action not observed when a larger amount of the drug and rapid intravenous infusion of the medication were used (Morton and Thomas, 1958). Such considerations are important in determining the appropriate dose of atropine in the various cardiac syndromes in which it may be of benefit, e.g., bradycardia (slow heart rate) associated with acute myocardial infarction, syncope, and bradycardia associated with a hyperactive carotid sinus reflex.

This excursion through two thousand or more years of the medical and social history of the belladonna drugs and the plants in which they are found is well summed up in a quotation from an article by Fred Kilmer of more than sixty years ago entitled "Rambling among the nightshades":

> The importance of these plants [the nightshades] through the centuries stands as a great fact in history. Starting at the beginning of things, and roaming here and there through the ages, we find that "much has been written, much forgotten, and but little is really known." We never arrive at the end. But even a haphazard ramble among these important drug plants is a pleasant, and may become a useful task.
>
> To the younger, or to the older, student of drugs, the lesson seems to be that a desultory ramble through a group of drug plants, or even the study of a single plant, can become an interesting pastime. But beyond this is the fact that in the realm of drugs there are still worlds waiting for the conqueror [1925, p. 38].

12

Diuretics: From Flies to Furosemide

THE Hearst Medical Papyrus of 1550 B.C. records early Egyptian mixtures and preparations "for causing one to urinate" (Leake, 1952, p. 82) and "to expel fluid accumulations from the body (and) from the heart" (p. 84). Over a thousand years later, Hippocrates commented in detail upon the management of patients with dropsy (an abnormal accumulation of fluid in the body) in his work *On Regimen in Acute Diseases*:

> There are two kinds of dropsy, the one anasarca, which, when formed is incurable; the other is accompanied with emphysema (tympanites?) and requires much good fortune to enable one to triumph over it. Laborious exertion, fomentation, and abstinence (are to be enjoined). The patient should eat dry and acrid things, for thus will he pass the more water, and his strength be kept up. If he labours under difficulty of breathing, if it is the summer season, and if he is in the prime of life, and is strong, blood should be abstracted from the arm, and then he should eat hot pieces of bread, dipped in dark wine and oil, drink very little, and labour much, and live on well-fed pork, boiled with vinegar, so that he may be able to endure hard exercises [c. 400 B.C., pp. 330–331].

Later in the same text, Hippocrates described the following preparation:

> A *draught for a dropsical person.* Take three cantharides [insects], and removing their head, feet, and wings, triturate their bodies in three cupfuls (cyathi) of water, and when the person who has drunk the draught complains of pain, let him have hot fomentations applied. The patient should be first anointed with oil, should take the draught fasting, and eat hot bread with oil [p. 333].

These excerpts suggest that Hippocrates may have recognized some of the different causes of fluid retention including that due to cardiopulmonary disease. Restriction of fluid intake, the use of alcoholic beverages with their known ability to produce a diuresis (an increased flow of urine), the suggestion that specific foods be eaten to the exclusion of others, and the reference to removal of blood—all have their modern therapeutic counterparts. More than two thousand years after Hippocrates made his recommendations, pharmacology texts of the nineteenth century still mentioned cantharides, known as *Cantharis vesicatoria*, the Spanish fly, for use as a diuretic (Biddle, 1880, pp. 388–390) or as an aphrodisiac (Bartholow, 1882, p. 609).

In retracing the early development of diuretic therapy, three medications warrant discussion—calomel, digitalis, and squill. Calomel (mercurous chloride) was employed by Paracelsus in the sixteenth century as a diuretic, although his application of the metal for this purpose seemed to have been either forgotten or overlooked (deStevens, 1963, p. 36).

In the late eighteenth century, William Withering (1785), in one of the classics of medical lore, recounted how his "opinion was asked concerning a family receipt for the cure of the dropsy. I was told that it had long been kept a secret by an old woman in Shropshire, who had sometimes made cures after the more regular practitioners had failed" (1785, p. 2). Later in the same text, Withering added: "It was in the course of this year [1775] that I began to use the Digitalis in dropsical cases" (p. 11). Since Withering's famous publication on digitalis is frequently referred to by only the first few words of the title, it may not always be remembered that a prime concern of the author was to describe the treatment of dropsy, as the full name of the work indicates—*An Account of the Foxglove, and Some of its Medical Uses: with Practical Remarks on Dropsy, and Other Diseases.* Squill, the bulb of a plant found on the shores of the Mediterranean, had been recognized many years earlier in ancient and medieval therapies as having similar properties for treating dropsy (Stannard, 1974). Withering mentioned squill in his report (1785, p. 3), pharmacology texts by Biddle (1880, pp. 295–296) and by Bartholow (1882, pp. 602–604) described the diuretic effects and medical uses of this medication in detail, and as recently as the 1940s Paul Dudley White recommended squill as a substitute for digitalis "in the very few cases who need digitalis but cannot take it because of a hypersensitive reaction or very strong prejudice against the taste" (1944, p. 779).

Editorials in medical publications during the late nineteenth century (*The Medical News*, 1887, 1888) reviewed several European articles describing the benefits of calomel therapy in patients with heart failure and fluid retention, with one of the earliest and best known being the report by Jendrássik of Budapest. Even before this information appeared, however, physicians were already administering combinations of calomel, digitalis leaf, and squill in their prescriptions, at times as a single pill. An article from Guy's Hospital in London is perhaps of more than usual interest in that the author refers to the use of such therapy by the well-known Thomas Addison (of pernicious anemia and adrenal gland insufficiency fame):

> It is of great importance, then, to relieve this distension, and it is most effectually done by the means already indicated, namely, by diuretics and by purgatives. A very favorite combination of my late senior colleague Dr. Addison consisted of a grain of calomel, a grain of powdered digitalis, and a grain of powdered squill, given night and morning for several days. These remedies act powerfully upon the whole of the abdominal glands; free bilious evacuation takes place, a larger quantity of urine is excreted, and the venous distension is greatly lessened, and secondarily the right side of the heart is relieved of its excessive fulness [Habershon, 1866, p. 309].

In the years that followed, a variety of pills composed of different proportions of calomel, digitalis leaf, and squill became available, at times named after an institution or well-known physician, e.g., Guy's Pills, Baillie's Pills, Addison's Pills, Niemeyer's Pills. Such medications remained in popular use through the early years of the twentieth century, having established, according to Rolleston, "a deserved reputation" (1909, p. 537).

The wide-ranging medical properties of tea were recognized hundreds of years ago, particularly in the Orient. Thus, it was not surprising that when tea reached England during the mid-seventeenth century, auction posters proclaimed its medical uses and virtues for the following purposes:

> Headache, Stone, Gravel, Dropsy, Scurvy, Sleepiness, Loss of Memory, Looseness or Gripping of the Guts, Heavy Dreams and Collick proceeding from Wind. Taken with Virgin's Honey instead of sugar, tea cleanses the Kidneys and Uterus and with Milk and Water it prevents consumption: if you are of corpulent body it ensures good Appetite, and if you have had a surfeit is just the thing to give you a gentle vomit [Maitland, 1982, p. 37].

In the late nineteenth and early twentieth centuries, xanthine derivatives were found to be responsible for the diuretic activity of both tea and coffee, with Koschlakoff and later Schroeder identifying caffeine as the active diuretic component in coffee, and Minkowski showing that theophylline in tea was an even more potent diuretic than caffeine (deStevens, 1963, p. 12). A combination of theobromine and sodium salicylate known as diuretin was developed during the last few years of the nineteenth century, described shortly thereafter in *The Extra Pharmacopoeia of Martindale and Westcott* as "a white powder, freely soluble in water. Is diuretic, without affecting nervous system and causing sleeplessness" (Martindale and Westcott, 1904, pp. 503–504). Diuretin maintained its role as a diuretic in the treatment of congestive heart failure for many years and was discussed as such by Paul Dudley White (1944, p. 782) and Paul Wood (1956, p. 303) in their well-known textbooks of cardiology.

Many other assorted agents were also used during the nineteenth century to increase urine flow, a partial listing of which includes the bitartrate and acetate of potassium, Indian hemp, dandelion, juniper, carrot seed, buchu, copaiba (the juice of a South American tree), garlic, parsley-root, and the previously mentioned Spanish fly (Biddle, 1880; Bartholow, 1882). At times, the strangeness of these medications and the ability of patients to tolerate and even to survive them would appear to be a tribute more to the hardiness of the human race than to the wisdom and skill of the medical profession, as witness this prescription: "Under the name of *cider mixture*, a compound infusion is used in dropsy, of which the following is the formula: Juniper berries, mustard seed, and ginger, each half an ounce; horseradish, parsley-root, each an ounce; cider, two pints—dose, a wineglassful, two or three times a day" (Biddle, 1880, p. 305). Fortunately, other diuretics were soon to be available.

Serendipidity was to play a major role in a discovery that revolutionized diuretic therapy and the care of patients with heart failure. In 1919, while a student at the Wenckebach Clinic in Vienna, Alfred Vogl observed that a nonedematous patient being treated for syphilis experienced a diuresis following injections of a mercurial compound called Novasurol. Subsequent administration of the drug to both syphilitic and nonsyphilitic patients with heart failure confirmed this increased production of urine. Many years later, reminiscing about this event, Vogl wrote:

> It became apparent that we were dealing with a potent diuretic which was independent of antisyphilitic activity and vastly superior to any diuretic thus far used. . . .
>
> This is the story of how a series of fortunate errors and coincidences resulted in "a discovery that has completely revolutionized the treatment of congestive heart failure" (Willius and Dry). The main credit should probably be given to the diligent nurse who, without specific orders, faithfully collected and charted the daily urine output. We may perhaps take pride in having taken note of an occurrence which had undoubtedly annoyed numerous patients who had received Novasurol injections in the preceding seven years (and whose complaints about polyuria were probably lightly dismissed by the physicians) [1950, p. 883].

After Vogl left the clinic, Saxl and Heilig continued these investigations, publishing their results in 1920 (Vogl, 1950). In later years, other studies indicated that the mercurial diuretics acted by decreasing the reabsorption of sodium and of chloride from the renal tubules (Blumgart, Gilligan, Levy, Brown, and Volk, 1934). Progress was made in reducing the toxicity of these drugs, in lessening their irritating effects at the site of injection, and in enhancing their diuretic action by combining them with mercaptan or theophylline. Administered either intramuscularly or intravenously for greatest effectiveness, the mercurial diuretics—mersalyl, mercuhydrin, mercaptomerin, among others—were the mainstays of diuretic therapy for 30–40 years following their accidental and fortunate discovery for this purpose in the course of treating patients with syphilis.

During the first half of the twentieth century, other diuretic agents were occasionally found to be useful. Urea was administered as an osmotic diuretic for edema of diverse etiologies. Ammonium chloride, although described as a diuretic in its own right, was used principally to potentiate the action of the mercurial diuretics and to prevent electrolyte difficulties associated with the latter. Nephrotic edema was treated with acacia until replaced by steroid therapy. During the 1950s, the diuretic action of a carbonic anhydrase inhibitor called acetazolamide was described; eventually this medication found its most useful application in the management of glaucoma.

William Schwartz in Boston was aware of previous work demonstrating that sulfanilamide, a drug used in the treatment of bacterial infections, had the ability to block or inhibit the action of the enzyme called carbonic anhydrase. Administering this medication to patients with heart failure in an attempt to promote a diuresis, he described his results as follows:

> Evidence indicating that sulfanilamide is capable of producing an increased sodium, potassium and water excretion in patients with congestive heart failure is presented. It appears that the inhibition of carbonic anhydrase in the cells of the renal tubules is responsible for this phenomenon. Other sulfonamides that are also inhibitors of carbonic anhydrase are under investigation in an effort to find a compound less toxic than sulfanilamide [Schwartz, 1949, p. 177].

With this background, investigators attempted to synthesize other compounds that might promote salt excretion and a diuresis. A new type of sulfonamide compound having a benzothiadiazine nucleus was developed by Novello and Sprague (1957). Chlorothiazide, the first of this new class of drugs to be widely used, initiated a new era not only in diuretic therapy but also in the treatment of hypertension. The "effective partnership of chemistry and biology" (Beyer, 1977, p. 410) that gave birth to this important discovery earned Novello, Sprague, Baer, and Beyer the 1975 Albert Lasker Special Public Health Award.

Since the introduction of the thiazides, ethacrynic acid and furosemide have been developed as even more potent medications, such drugs now forming the cornerstone of present-day diuretic therapy. Potassium-sparing preparations, namely spironolactone, triamterene, and amiloride, are used in combination with these saluretic agents. To these modern-day diuretics can be added those drugs that may contribute to a diuresis through their hemodynamic impact on the venous and arterial circulation and on the heart—the vasodilators and angiotensin-converting enzyme inhibitors. From flies to furosemide, from calomel to captopril—it has been a long and interesting journey.

13

Vitamin B$_{12}$ and Pernicious Anemia: Stomach and Bone Marrow—An Odd Couple

THE discovery of vitamin B$_{12}$ had to wait 100 years while the secrets of pernicious anemia were slowly being unraveled. An initial step toward understanding this disease might well have been taken when Dr. Combe of Edinburgh speculated with amazing foresight upon a fatal case of anemia: "for it is probably owing to some disorder of the digestive and assimilative organs, that its characteristic symptom [the anemia] has its origin, and to the correction of this derangement, we must look for a removal of the disease" (1824, p. 204). The classic description of what would eventually be called pernicious anemia has been attributed to the famous Thomas Addison of Guy's Hospital, London, who wrote:

> For a long period I had from time to time met with a very remarkable form of general anaemia, occurring without any discoverable cause whatever; cases in which there had been no previous loss of blood, no exhausting diarrhoea, no chlorosis, no purpura, no renal, splenic, miasmatic, glandular, strumous, or malignant disease. Accordingly, in speaking of this form of anaemia in clinical lecture, I, perhaps with little propriety, applied to it the term "idiopathic," to distinguish it from cases in which there existed more or less evidence of some of the usual causes or concomitants of the anaemic state [1855, p. 2].

It is interesting that none of the clinical stigmata often associated with pernicious anemia such as glossitis, neurologic changes, or jaundice were mentioned, and that the description of the anemia appears to be almost incidental to Addison's discussion of the adrenal disease that would eventually also be named after him.

97

Several years later, Samuel Fenwick of London Hospital described the findings at postmortem examination in a fatal case of Addisonian anemia:

> The whole of the glandular structure of the organ [stomach] was in a state of atrophy: in no part could I succeed in procuring a section of normal tissue. . . .
> It is well known that an infusion of the [normal] gastric mucous membrane, when mixed with dilute hydrochloric acid, will dissolve albuminous substances. . . . I carefully scraped off the mucous membrane from the splenic and middle regions of the stomach of the preceding case, and infused it in two ounces of distilled water along with half a drachm of hydrochloric acid for twelve hours. A cube of hard-boiled white of egg, fifteen grains in weight, was then digested for nine hours at blood-heat; but at the end of this period the albumen had not lost in weight, and the only change produced was a slight softening on its surface. This experiment, therefore, confirmed the conclusion derived from microscopical examination, that the gland-structure of the stomach had been so seriously diseased that it could not have been capable of performing its functions during life [1870, p. 79].

Lack of hydrochloric acid in the stomach contents of a patient with Addisonian anemia during life was documented by Cahn and von Mering (1886), an observation subsequently used for many years as a diagnostic test in establishing the diagnosis. Thus, increasing evidence was being accumulated linking the stomach with this form of anemia.

As cited by Huser (1966), fifteen cases of a previously unknown form of anemia were described by Biermer of Zurich in 1872—"Über eine Form von progressiver perniciöser Anämie." This term used by Biermer—pernicious anemia—has since that time been applied to Addisonian idiopathic anemia.

That certain blood diseases might be related to nutritional deficiencies was often suspected but never clearly proved. However, during the early years of the twentieth century, it was established with certainty that the anemia of chronically bled dogs could be corrected with a variety of food products, including liver (Whipple, Robscheit, and Hooper, 1920). Elders, having observed that a patient with pernicious anemia responded to a diet similar to one he had used successfully in treating cases of sprue in the Dutch East Indies—underdone horse-meat, milk, cod-liver oil, eggs, and fruits—concluded:

> Sprue and pernicious anaemia have so much in common that it is difficult to accept a different aetiology for the two diseases. If they have the same aetiology it is most probable that pernicious anemia is, like sprue, a deficiency disease,

and as such should be curable, or at least amenable to improvement by well-chosen food [1925, p. 77].

The results of this and other similar studies linking pernicious anemia to the nutritional deficiencies culminated in the historic paper by George R. Minot and William P. Murphy of Boston entitled "Treatment of pernicious anemia by a special diet" (Figure 13.1):

> The dietetic treatment of pernicious anemia is of more importance than hitherto generally recognized.
> Forty-five patients with pernicious anemia observed essentially in sequence are continuing to take a special diet that they have now been living on for from about six weeks to two years but which was temporarily omitted by three. This diet is composed especially of food rich in complete proteins and iron—particularly liver—and containing an abundance of fruits and fresh vegetables and relatively low in fat.
> Following the diet, all the patients showed a prompt, rapid and distinct remission of their anemia, coincident with at least marked symptomatic improvement [1926, pp. 475–476].

It was further stated: "We are inclined to believe that something contained in the foods rich in complete proteins is particularly responsible for the improvement in the state of the blood" (p. 475). In 1934, Minot and Murphy, together with Whipple, received the Nobel Prize for Medicine for their pioneering contributions.

Starting in the late 1920s and building upon these observations, William Castle undertook additional studies of pernicious anemia and liver therapy at the Thorndike Memorial Laboratory in Boston, trying to understand this disease and searching for the "something" in food described by Minot and Murphy (1926, p. 475). The question was raised by Castle

> as to why normal persons did not need to eat a half-pound of liver a day in order to stave off pernicious anemia. The primary, outstanding and apparently irremediable difference between the normal individual and the patient with pernicious anemia, whether developed spontaneously or as a result of gastrectomy, seemed to be a lack of gastric secretion. How was it that the stomach of the normal person could derive something from ordinary food that was for him equivalent to eating liver? With these thoughts in mind, it did not require much sagacity to imagine that "by substituting some digestive process of the normal stomach . . . it might be possible to affect the patient's disease favorably" [1961, pp. 66–67].

Years later, in reviewing the results of many experiments, Castle (1961) noted that the stomachs of patients with pernicious anemia

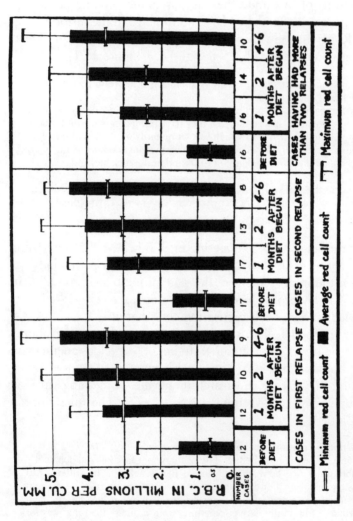

Fig. 13.1. A graphic representation from the landmark article by Minot and Murphy (1926) demonstrating improvement in the red blood cell counts of patients with pernicious anemia who were treated with special diets. *Source:* Minot, G. R., & Murphy, W. P. (1926), Treatment of pernicious anemia by a special diet. *J. Amer. Med. Assn.,* 87:470–476. Copyright 1926, American Medical Association.

were deficient in a specific secretion, called "intrinsic factor." The presence of this secretion in the stomach of normal people permitted absorption of enough anti-pernicious anemia substance ("extrinsic factor") from ordinary foods to prevent anemia. However, lacking the "intrinsic factor," patients with pernicious anemia could only obtain adequate amounts of this anti-pernicious anemia substance by ingesting massive amounts of a food, such as liver, that was rich in the latter material. Thus, the link between the stomach and anemia foretold by Combe (1824) over 100 years earlier was now defined and the door was open to rational, specific therapy.

In the two decades that followed the work of Minot and Murphy (1926), an intensive search was undertaken by many investigators to isolate and identify this "extrinsic factor" (Castle, 1961, p. 56). Finally, a group of scientists headed by Karl Folkers at Merck Research Laboratories in New Jersey reported: "Further purification of clinically active liver fractions has led to the isolation, in minute amounts, of a crystalline compound which is highly active for the growth of *L. lactis*. This compound is being called vitamin B$_{12}$" (Rickes, Brink, Koniuszy, Wood, and Folkers, 1948, p. 396). Experiments being conducted almost simultaneously in England by Smith and Parker were similarly successful in purifying this "anti-pernicious anaemia factor" (1948, p. viii). Soon thereafter, Randolph West at Columbia University confirmed that "Crystalline vitamin B$_{12}$ has shown positive hematological activity in three cases of addisonian pernicious anemia" (1948, p. 398). A few years later, the structural formula of vitamin B$_{12}$, called cyanocobalamin, was determined by a process called x-ray crystallography, the investigators commenting that the "molecule that appears is very beautifully composed, not far from spherical in form, with all the more chemically reactive groups on its surface" (Hodgkin, Kamper, Mackay, Pickworth, Trueblood, and White, 1956, p. 65).

The combined efforts of many from various medical disciplines had led to the cure of a previously fatal disease. Thus, therapy for pernicious anemia, initially consisting of the daily ingestion of half a pound of liver, had been successfully, and mercifully, reduced to treatment with a few micrograms of intramuscular vitamin B$_{12}$ every few weeks.

Until the early years of the twentieth century, pernicious anemia was usually a fatal illness. Its cure, first with liver in 1926 by Minot and Murphy and then with vitamin B$_{12}$, has been one of the major triumphs of medical research in the present century. As so well phrased by William Castle, a modern-day hero in the conquest of this disease, "her [nature's] foreclosure of the mortgages on the lives of the tenants of this disorder has become rare since 1926" [1953, p. 603].

14

Insulin: The Internal Secretion of the Pancreas

THE Greek physician Aretaeus the Cappadocian, in one of the earliest accounts of diabetes, described it as follows:

> Diabetes is a wonderful affection, not very frequent among men, being a melting down of the flesh and limbs into urine. Its cause is of a cold and humid nature, as in dropsy. The course is the common one, namely, the kidneys and bladder; for the patients never stop making water, but the flow is incessant, as if from the opening of aqueducts. The nature of the disease, then, is chronic, and it takes a long period to form; but the patient is short-lived, if the constitution of the disease be completely established; for the melting is rapid, the death speedy. Moreover, life is disgusting and painful; thirst, un-quenchable; excessive drinking, which, however is disproportionate to the large quantity of urine, for more urine is passed; and one cannot stop them either from drinking or making water. Or if for a time they abstain from drinking, their mouth becomes parched and their body dry. . . .
> . . . Hence, the disease appears to me to have got the name of *diabetes*, as if from the Greek word . . . (*which signifies a siphon*), because the fluid does not remain in the body, but uses the man's body as a ladder . . . whereby to leave it [Aretaeus, *c.* 120–200 A.D., pp. 338–339].

This description by Aretaeus is consistent with that of patients with diabetes mellitus, although without appropriate diagnostic procedures, it would not have been possible for him to clearly differentiate these cases from those with similar symptoms due to other less common causes, e.g., diabetes insipidus.

According to Major, Susruta, the great surgeon of ancient Hindu medicine, stated that the perspiration and expectoration of patients with diabetes "acquire a sweet taste and smell like that of honey" (1954a, p. 70). Several centuries later, Thomas Willis commented that the urine of diabetic patients "was wonderfully sweet as it were imbued with Honey or Sugar" (1679, p. 192), an observation confirmed almost a hundred years later when, by evaporating urine from diabetic patients, Mathew Dobson proved that it did indeed contain sugar (Dobson, 1776).

Further progress in understanding and treating diabetes occurred in 1869 when Paul Langerhans described the pancreatic islets, small clusters of cells of unusual appearance within the body of the pancreas (Murray, 1969). Twenty years later, in an epoch-making publication entitled "Diabetes mellitus after extirpation of the pancreas," Joseph von Mering and Oskar Minkowski of Strassburg University demonstrated that diabetes could be produced in a dog by removing the pancreas—a pancreatectomy:

> As far as the results of extirpation of the pancreas are concerned, we have already mentioned the most important: *After complete removal of the organ, the dogs became diabetic.* It has not to do simply with a transient glycosuria, but a genuine *lasting diabetes mellitus,* which in every respect corresponds to the most severe form of this disease in man [1889, p. 205].

On the basis of such observations, several investigators began to speculate whether there may exist a relationship between diabetes and the islet cells described by Langerhans. Edward Schäfer wrote:

> The only fact that appears certain in connection with the manner in which the pancreas prevents excessive production of sugar within the body is that this effect must be produced by the formation of some material secreted internally by the gland, and probably by the interstitial vascular islets, and that this internally secreted material profoundly modifies the carbohydrate metabolism of the tissues [1895, p. 342].

Eugene Lindsay Opie, while an instructor in pathology at the Johns Hopkins University, described the presence of hyaline degeneration and destruction of the islets of Langerhans in patients with diabetes, again suggesting that these cells might be the source of the internal secretion that was lacking in this disease (1901).

With this background, the search now focused on finding the antidiabetic substance within the pancreas. In 1908, Zülzer reported that he had successfully reduced the amount of sugar in the urine of an experimental animal with an intravenously injected pancreatic extract (Murray, 1969). However, supplies of this material were limited, and impurities caused fever and other toxicities when the extract was injected into humans. Although a pharmaceutical firm appeared interested in the potential therapeutic value of this study, the project was later discontinued (Murray, 1969).

During this period, Ernest Lyman Scott, a graduate student in the Department of Physiology at the University of Chicago, reasoned that previous difficulties in identifying an antidiabetic substance may have been due to its destruction by digestive enzymes of the pancreas during the extraction procedure (1911–1912). In an attempt to inactivate these enzymes and prevent this destructive process from occurring, Scott exposed fresh adult animal pancreas to alcohol. Aqueous extracts of this preparation were then injected into diabetic dogs, resulting in a significant decrease in the urinary excretion of sugar. However, Scott cautiously questioned whether this effect may have been related to a temperature elevation or to nonspecific toxic effects, suggesting that these issues needed to be resolved before it could be claimed that his extract truly contained an active antidiabetic principle.

In the meantime, other experiments were being performed by the well-known Rumanian physiologist Nicolas Paulesco in which dog pancreas was minced and mixed with distilled water, stored in ice for 24 hours, then filtered and 0.7 gm. sodium chloride per 100 ml added (Murray, 1971). When injected into the veins of diabetic dogs, blood sugar and urinary sugar and acetone levels fell. Paulesco's work demonstrating these effects of his pancreatic extract was interrupted by World War I, and it was not until 1921 that his results were published—"Recherche sur le rôle du pancréas dans l'assimilation nutritive" and "Influence de la quantité de pancréas employée pour préparer l'extrait injecté dans le sang chez un animal diabétique" (Murray, 1971). Before problems of purification and large-scale production could be resolved, rapidly occurring events in Canada and the United States had already led to the clinical availability of insulin, and Paulesco's studies were largely overlooked.

It is evident from this brief survey that although the world would later recognize, remember, and pay tribute to others for the discovery of insulin, much work had already been accomplished in this field and several earlier investigators may well have been entitled to a share of the honor of discovering it.

Frederic Grant Banting provided the leadership, enthusiasm, and determination that guided the final steps leading to the discovery and clinical use of insulin. Banting, an orthopedic surgeon, had settled in London, Ontario, after serving in the Canadian army. While working part-time as a demonstrator in the physiology department at the local university, he became interested in diabetes after reading an article in which it was suggested that the islets of Langerhans may be responsible for secreting a hormone affecting carbohydrate metabolism. Banting conceived the idea that by ligating the pancreatic duct and causing atrophy of alveolar cells (an approach that had been tried before), an extract of the remaining tissue could be obtained that would be effective in pancreatectomized dogs (Murray, 1969; Bliss, 1982).

Banting presented his ideas to John Macleod, Professor of Physiology at the University of Toronto. An assistant was obtained with a background in biochemistry, Charles Best, a student recently trained by Macleod in a micro-method for measuring blood sugar levels in small quantities of blood. Experiments commenced in May 1921. As in the earlier attempts of others, the pancreatic ducts of dogs were tied in order to cause degeneration of cells containing the digestive enzymes, and by so doing, prevent destruction of the antidiabetic substance during the extraction process. As then described by Banting and Best, "The degenerated pancreas was swiftly removed, and sliced into a chilled mortar containing Ringer's solution. The mortar was placed in freezing mixture and the contents partially frozen. The half frozen gland was then completely macerated. The solution was filtered . . . and the filtrate . . . injected intravenously [into dogs]" (1922, p. 254). It was later discovered that pancreatic duct ligation was actually unnecessary for isolating the antidiabetic principle, and that exposure to acid alcohol, as described previously by Scott, could inhibit the destructive action of the digestive enzyme-producing cells. Banting and Best called the material they had isolated isletin, although this was subsequently changed to the previously recommended name of insulin (Murray, 1969).

Results of these experiments were presented at the American Physiological Society Meetings in New Haven in December 1921. The following year, a landmark article appeared—"The internal secretion of the pancreas"—containing this carefully written statement:

> In the course of our experiments we [Banting and Best] have administered over seventy-five doses of extract from degenerated pancreatic tissue to ten different diabetic animals. Since the extract has always produced a reduction of the percentage sugar of the blood and of the sugar excreted in the urine, we feel justified in stating that this extract contains the internal secretion of the pancreas [Banting and Best, 1922, p. 265].

Dogs were kept alive indefinitely with these injections i.e., for 70 days, with animals such as Marjorie becoming well-known for their participation in these experiments (Best, 1972). During this period, John Collip, biochemist, joined the Toronto team and was a major contributor in helping to prepare insulin of sufficient potency and purity for clinical use. The excitement of these times, the details of these experiments, and the personal and professional differences between the participants, have been previously recorded in their own words (Best, 1972; Macleod, 1978; Bliss, 1982).

It has been over sixty-five years since an initial group of seven patients received pancreatic extract obtained by these investigators in Toronto (Banting, Best, Collip, Campbell, and Fletcher, 1922). These precedent-shattering conclusions were asserted in their report:

> (1). Blood sugar can be markedly reduced even to the normal values.
> (2). Glycosuria can be abolished.
> (3). The acetone bodies can be made to disappear from the urine.
> (4). The respiratory quotient shows evidence of increased utilization of carbohydrates.
> (5). A definite improvement is observed in the general condition of these patients and in addition the patients themselves report a subjective sense of well being and increased vigor for a period following the administration of these preparations [1922, p. 146].

Another diabetic patient, a five-year-old boy, was treated by Banting a few months after this report, receiving his first insulin injection on July 10, 1922. The patient, still alive and taking insulin sixty-six years later in 1988, was said at the time to have received the injections for a longer period than any one else in the world (Wardner, 1988).

Banting and Best gave the patent rights for the insulin-producing process to Toronto University. The information was then made available to Eli Lilly and Company of Indianapolis, where a chemist, George Walden, devised a method of purification by isoelectric fractionation. The yield and potency of material from animal preparations were improved, large-scale production became possible, and within a year or two, insulin was available for clinical use at various institutions. The significance of this work was recognized with the presentation of the Nobel Prize in Medicine to Banting and Macleod in 1923 (but strangely not to Best). Shortly thereafter, a clash of personalities resulted in the break-up of this world-famous research team (Murray, 1969; Bliss, 1982).

Much has since happened in the development of insulin and treatment of diabetes. Pure crystalline insulin was obtained by John Abel of Johns Hopkins University (1926). Longer-acting preparations requiring less frequent injections—i.e., protamine zinc insulin, the Lente insulins—became available. During the 1950s, Frederick Sanger of Cambridge University worked out the sequence of the amino acids and the disulfide linkages that make up the insulin molecule, receiving the Nobel Prize for Chemistry in 1958 for this work (Sanger, 1960). Oral hypoglycemic agents for treating diabetes, insulin pumps, and biologically engineered human insulin are more recent extensions of the insulin story.

Diabetes is now a manageable disease: insulin therapy has saved countless lives and allowed many people to participate in activities that would otherwise have not been possible. However, to be a diabetic and to be treated with insulin continues to give rise to formidable physical and emotional problems, in which the balance between patient, disease, and therapeutic efforts is ever delicate, as these excerpts from the poem "Diabetes" by the contemporary American poet James Dickey record so vividly (1970, pp. 8–9):

> My eyes are green as lettuce with my diet,
> My weight is down,
> One pocket nailed with needles and injections, the other dragging
> With sugar cubes to balance me in life
> And hold my blood
> Level, level. Tell me, black riders, does this do any good?
> Tell me what I need to know about my time
> In the world. O out of the fiery
>
> Furnace of pine-woods, in the sap-smoke and crownfire of needles,
> Say when I'll die. When will the sugar rise boiling
> Against me, and my brain be sweetened
> to death?
> *In heavy summer, like this day.*
> All right! Physicians, witness! I will shoot my veins
> Full of insulin. Let the needle burn
> In.

15

Oxygen: The Eminently Respirable Air

MORE than three hundred years ago, Robert Boyle (1627–1691) at Oxford demonstrated that an animal could not survive and that sulfur would not burn in a vacuum, thus establishing that air is necessary for both life and combustion (Cournand, 1964, p. 32). A few years later, Richard Lower investigated the reason for the difference in color between arterial and venous blood, edging toward identifying the specific substance in air responsible for Boyle's observations. The results of Lower's studies, among the most significant in the history of medicine and physiology, are contained in his *Tractatus de Corde* in the chapter entitled "The movement and colour of the blood," the concluding comments of which state:

> On this account it is extremely probable that the blood takes in air in its course through the lungs, and owes it bright colour entirely to the admixture of air. Moreover, after the air has in large measure left the blood again within the body and the parenchyma of the viscera, and has transpired through the pores of the body, it is equally consistent with reason that the venous blood, which has lost its air, should forthwith appear darker and blacker.
>
> From this it is easy to imagine the great advantage accruing to the blood from the admixture of air, and the great importance attaching to the air taken in being always healthy and pure; one can see, too, how greatly in error are those, who altogether deny this intercourse of air and blood. Without such intercourse, any one would be able to live in as good health in the stench of a prison as among the most pleasant vegetation. Wherever, in a word, a fire can burn sufficiently well, there we can equally well breathe [Lower, 1669, pp. 170–171].

Written with simplicity and clarity, this extraordinary work, as noted by Cournand, established "that the function of the pulmonary circulation is the arterialization of the venous blood" (1964, pp. 33–34). These historic observations paved the way for later studies of the composition of air itself. During the years 1774–1775, a Presbyterian minister and self-taught chemist in Leeds, Joseph Priestley, prepared a gas by heating mercurous red oxide in a closed container, noting that a candle placed in this gas "burned . . . with remarkably vigorous flame" (Cournand, 1964, p. 41), and that mice lived longer in a container filled with this new substance than when breathing equal volumes of atmospheric air. This gas, eventually to be known as oxygen, was initially called *dephlogisticated air*. Priestley, unpopular with the public because of his liberal political and religious views and his support of the American colonists and the French revolution, eventually left England to join his sons in Pennsylvania.

Antoine Laurent Lavoisier (1743–1794), an exceptional and gifted man of many talents, lived all his life in Paris as a successful financier, politician, and scientist. In 1777, he presented an essay at the Academy of Sciences entitled *Experiments on the respiration of animals and on the changes affecting air in its passage through the lungs*, concluding with the following observations:

> Eminently respirable air that enters the lung, leaves it in the form of chalky aeriform acid $[CO_2]$ . . . in almost equal volume. . . .
> Respiration only acts on the portion of pure air that is eminently respirable . . . the excess, that is, its mephitic portion [nitrogen], is a purely passive medium which enters and leaves the lungs . . . without change or alteration.
> The respirable portion of air has the property to combine with blood and its combination results in its red color [Cournand, 1964, p. 46].

Lavoisier is generally credited with establishing the principle of respiratory gas exchange as it is presently understood, having drawn inspiration for some of his ideas from a knowledge of Priestley's work (Cournand, 1964, p. 44). Tragically, like Priestley, he too was a victim of his times, with his path unfortunately leading in 1794 to the guillotine of the French revolution rather than to America. A contemporary, hearing of Lavoisier's untimely death, uttered these well-known words: "It took only one moment to sever that head, and perhaps a century will not be enough to produce another like it" (Cournand, 1964, p. 43).

The identification and isolation of oxygen and other gases aroused considerable interest in their potential medical uses. Thomas Beddoes, a graduate from the medical department of Oxford University, established the short-lived Pneumatic Institution of Clifton in 1798 (Miller, 1931). There, gases were prepared and equipment invented for treating a wide variety of medical problems, as outlined by Beddoes and Watt in a series of publications entitled *Considerations on the Medicinal Use, and on the Production of Factitious Airs* (1796). Unfortunately, the application of oxygen and inhalation therapy for such a diversity of diseases without a sound understanding of pathophysiological principles led to many therapeutic failures and the eventual closure of the institute. For his creative efforts, however, Beddoes has since been regarded as a pioneer and innovator in the field of inhalation therapy. Of tangential historical interest to the Pneumatic Institution itself are two men who worked there with Beddoes and who later had outstanding careers of their own—James Watt of steam engine fame, and Humphry Davy, discoverer, while working with Beddoes, of the anesthetic properties of the gas nitrous oxide and inventor of the safety lamp for coal miners.

Throughout the nineteenth century, inhalation therapy continued to be employed somewhat indiscriminately in the treatment of a broad spectrum of diseases, prompting Tovell and Remlinger to comment about this period: "As a result of its [oxygen's] abuse and misuse, considerable skepticism arose as to its actual therapeutic value, and during the next hundred years [following the work of Beddoes] the procedures suffered from the unmerited neglect which eventually supervenes when a method is used as a panacea" (1941, p. 1939). In the early years of the twentieth century, however, rapid strides in understanding the physiology of respiration and in devising and utilizing better equipment changed the situation. A number of brilliant investigators, among them the outstanding group from Copenhagen of Christian Bohr, August Krogh, and K. A. Hasselbalch, laid the foundation for present-day therapy by precisely defining the relationships of oxygen and carbon dioxide in body fluids, performing vital experiments "in which the effects of CO_2 [carbon dioxide] tension on the binding of oxygen by hemoglobin was demonstrated, with a full set of oxygen dissociation curves at varying CO_2 tensions" (Cournand, 1964, p. 57). Important contributions concerning the physical chemistry of blood in relation to respiratory gases were made by the well-known physiologists John Scott Haldane and Joseph Barcroft in England, Lawrence Henderson and his associates at Harvard, and Donald

Van Slyke and his colleagues at the Rockefeller Institute in New York. Henderson commented upon the complex and fundamental relationship existing between electrolytes and gases in the blood and other tissues in his classic publication *Blood: A Study in General Physiology*, stating that

> the discovery by Christiansen, Douglas, and Haldane of the effect of oxygenation of blood upon its carbon dioxide dissociation curves finally led me to the conclusion which should have been drawn a decade earlier, that every one of the variables involved in the respiratory exchanges of blood must be a mathematical function of all the others [1928, pp. 95–96].

These vital studies into the physicochemical basis of alveolar-capillary gas exchange, to which so many capable investigators contributed, were concisely summed up by the Nobel laureate André Cournand:

> The final synthesis was Henderson's large nomogram upon which all the following were set forth: chloride concentration in plasma and cells, cell volume, per cent water in cells, base bound to protein, cell and plasma bicarbonate, total CO_2, CO_2 tension, plasma pH, cell pH, R.Q., oxygen tension, oxygen saturation, and hemoglobin concentration. As the blood moves from the pulmonary arterial to the pulmonary venous vessels in its passage through the lungs, uptake of oxygen renders hemoglobin more acid, and thus binds more potassium; bicarbonate, chloride, and water leave the cells; loss of CO_2 to the alveoli decreases bicarbonate both of plasma and cells; the plasma sodium can now accept the added chloride and bicarbonate from the cells; thus there is a minimum shift in plasma pH [1964, p. 62].

At the same time as the classical theories of respiratory physiology and of the interchange of gases between air and blood were being clarified, the clinical consequences of oxygen lack and of oxygen therapy were being defined, and procedures and equipment were being devised upon the basis of a sounder understanding of physiologic principles. Today's management of patients with respiratory problems owes much to the ingenuity and imagination of those involved during these early years as the field of respiratory care and oxygen therapy matured.

In 1912, Hürter showed that puncture of the radial artery was safe (Stadie, 1919). Seven years later, William Stadie at the Hospital of the Rockefeller Institute for Medical Research outlined the technique of arterial puncture as it was then being applied during a severe influenza epidemic. Oxygen content, oxygen capacity, and oxygen unsaturation determinations were performed on arterial blood of the patients, particularly those with pneumonia and cyanosis, using the well-known gasometric method of Van Slyke (1918). Although blood gas analysis has since become a much less cumbersome procedure, the technique of arterial puncture, an important tool in pulmonary medicine, has changed little since Stadie described it over seventy years ago.

In an effort to evaluate the physiologic and clinical consequences of oxygen deprivation, subjects, many times the investigators themselves, were exposed to experimental anoxia for varying periods of time (Haldane, Kellas, and Kennaway, 1919; Barcroft, Cooke, Hartridge, Parsons, and Parsons, 1920). The well-known physiologist Joseph Barcroft described his experiences living for several days in a glass respiration chamber in which the partial pressure of oxygen was gradually reduced as low as 45 mm. of mercury:

> Exploration of the condition of the arterial blood is only in its infancy, yet many cases have been recorded in which in illness the arterial blood has lacked oxygen as much as or more than my own did in the respiration chamber when I was lying on the last day, with occasional vomiting, racked with headache, and at times able to see clearly only as an effort of concentration. A sick man, if his blood is as anoxic as mine was, cannot be expected to fare better as the result, and so he may be expected to have all my troubles in addition to the graver ones which are, perhaps, attributable to some toxic cause. Can he be spared the anoxaemia? The result of our calculations, so far, points to the fact that the efficient way of combating the anoxic condition is to give oxygen [1920, p. 489].

Stadie, in addition to describing the previously mentioned technique of arterial puncture, demonstrated at the same time that "There is a definite relation between the degree of cyanosis and the per cent of arterial unsaturation" (1919, p. 238) in patients with pneumonia. Two years later, the harmful effects of cyanosis and anoxia were further examined by Jonathan Meakins, Professor of Therapeutics at the University of Edinburgh, who wrote:

> The animal organism may exist for a considerable time deprived of the ordinary means of nourishment, but a comparatively short and sudden starvation of a sufficient supply of oxygen to the tissues is fraught with very disastrous results. These ill effects are particularly evident in the impairment of the proper functions of the cardio-vascular, the nervous and the glandular systems. Therefore it is important that where anoxaemia develops it should, if possible, be relieved [1921, p. 79].

Meakins went on to describe oxygen treatment in patients with severe lobar pneumonia and cyanosis, noting that

[i]t is most important—perhaps the most important—factor in the treatment of pneumonia, apart from the specific cure of the infection, that the patient should be prevented from developing an anoxaemia, as represented by the cyanosis. The early administration of oxygen to such cases with cyanosis is most imperative, as there is great danger of being irretrievably too late when the signs of cardio-vascular paralysis appear [1921, p. 89].

At the same time as the medical conditions that might benefit from oxygen therapy were being evaluated, equipment and methods for oxygen administration were being designed. In the early years of the twentieth century, this initially took the form of simple nasal catheters. Prompted by the need to treat pulmonary edema resulting from gas poisoning during World War I, Haldane devised a face mask, commenting:

Existing methods of giving oxygen are nearly always very crude and wasteful of oxygen, and it is not possible to graduate efficiently the percentage of oxygen administered. The simple apparatus now to be described is designed to remedy these defects and render practically possible the prolonged administration of air enriched with as little oxygen as will suffice for the purpose aimed at [1917, p. 183].

During this same span of time, Meltzer (1917) described an oral insufflation method for administering oxygen, and Hill (1921) designed an oxygen tent to fit over the upper part of a patient when in bed. Stadie constructed an oxygen chamber

designed so that pneumonia patients with anoxemia may be placed in it and breathe an atmosphere containing 40 to 60 per cent of oxygen.
        4. The chamber is easy of ingress and egress, is economical in cost of operation, and comfortably accommodates patient and attendants so that adequate nursing and medical attention can be given at all times [1922, p. 335].

Alvan Barach, considered by many the father of modern-day oxygen and inhalation therapy, made many contributions to this field between the 1920s and 1940s. He not only provided a sounder understanding of oxygen use and equipment but also was instrumental in establishing many basic guidelines and standards of care for administering inhalation therapy (Committee on Public Relations of the New York Academy of Medicine, 1943). Several types of masks, oxygen chambers and tents, and predictable-dose devices were recommended, depending upon the availability of different materials and the ingenuity of those designing the equipment. On occasion, medical application of a device accompanied or followed its use for another purpose, as in the invention of a high-concentration oxygen mask for supplying oxygen to aviators at high altitudes, the BLB oxygen mask, by Boothby, Lovelace, and Bulbulian at the Mayo Clinic (Boothby, 1938; Lovelace, 1938; Bulbulian, 1938). These circumstances were similar to those which arose many years later when space program equipment was adapted for monitoring patients in critical care medicine.

Like most forms of treatment in medicine, oxygen therapy was not without possible side effects or toxicity. In an extensive review of oxygen poisoning, Stadie, Riggs, and Haugaard (1944) introduced their discussion by quoting a translated excerpt from Paul Bert's classic *La Pression Barometrique*, published in 1878: "One finds clearly demonstrated . . . the apparently paradoxical result that under the influence of very high oxygenation of the blood, the tissues oxidize less, organic combustions diminish in energy, production of CO_2, excretion of urine, the destruction of sugar in the blood are diminished, and that as a result temperature falls" (1944, pp. 84–85). At the close of the nineteenth century, Smith pointed out that "Oxygen which at the tension of the atmosphere stimulates the lung cells to active absorption, at a higher tension acts as an irritant, or pathological stimulant, and produces inflammation" (1899, p. 35).

The tragedy of retrolental fibroplasia and blindness in infants receiving high levels of oxygen at birth was described by Patz, Hoeck, and De La Cruz (1952), and reviewed by Howell and Ford (1985) in a chapter entitled "The Paradoxes of a Small American Disaster" from their book *Medical Mysteries*. The development of oxygen pneumonitis has been reported in patients on ventilators (Hyde and Rawson, 1969), serving as a reminder that oxygen therapy, like any other treatment, needs to be used with discrimination and with careful and constant monitoring.

Humble and self-evident as some of the observations by clinicians and respiratory physiologists over the last 300 years might now appear, from their experiences and knowledge have evolved the ability of present-day physicians to understand and use oxygen—the "eminently respirable air" of Lavoisier (Cournand, 1964, p. 46)—with care, with safety, and with maximal advantage and benefit for patients.

16

Leeches: The Medicinal Vampires

ONE of the more unusual methods of treatment recorded in the annals of medical history consists of the application of leeches to the skin in order to remove blood. The bizarreness attributed to this form of therapy may in part have been related to the folklore of vampires and the legends of Count Dracula. Over 2,000 years ago, during the classic period of Greek medicine, Nicander (Nikandros) of Colophon described the therapeutic use of leeches in his medical poem *Alexipharmaca* (Major, 1954a, p. 146). Since then, the leech has maintained a constant presence in medicine.

The medicinal leech (*Hirudo medicinalis*) is a green parasitic worm with brown stripes belonging to the class Hirudinea, distantly related to the earthworm, measuring from 5 to 10 centimeters in length at rest and up to twice that while the body is stretched when swimming; typically, it is found under stones in fresh-water ponds, streams, and marshes. The hind end terminates in a large muscular disc or sucker with which the leech can attach itself when crawling. A smaller sucker at the anterior end encloses an unusual mouth composed of three jaws, each with 60 to 100 teeth, and arranged in such a fashion that when attaching itself and cutting into flesh, a three-spoked radial incision is made, similar to a Mercedes-Benz logo. Weighing at times 2 to 3 grams, leeches can ingest amounts of blood at one sitting that may increase their initial weights as much as 800%; they can remain satiated for periods of up to several months (Payton, 1981b; Green and Gilby, 1983; Lent, 1985).

To the Anglo-Saxon of the Middle Ages, a physician was known as a leech, and treatment manuals and writings of these times were

known as leech books (Payton, 1981a). Tempting as it might be to
associate the name leech as applied to a physician with the parasitic
leech, both being involved as they are with blood, the literature does
not appear to relate the two. Still, how well this unusual physician's
assistant, this parasitic worm, has "attached" itself to man and has
fared through the ages is as much a testimony to the strange practices
of physicians as it is to the hardiness of the leech and the fortitude of
patients (Figure 16.1).

The employment of leeches during the Greco-Roman period was
described by Antyllos, said to be the greatest surgeon of antiquity
(Major, 1954a, p. 203), and by Galen (Mettler, 1947, p. 338). The
blood-sucking parasite continued its colorful journey through history,
as attested to by the observations and recommendations of Avicenna,
the author of the great source book of Arabian medicine of the middle
ages, A *Treatise on the Canon of Medicine*:

> 1038. The blood which leeches remove from the body comes from deeper
> down than that obtained by wet cupping. . . .
> 1040. *Site of application*—The place where the leeches are to be applied
> must be . . . well laved with nitre-water and rubbed till red. Dry carefully. Dip
> the leeches in fresh tepid water. . . . The point of application may be smeared
> with clay (or moistened with sugar-water or milk) or scratched with a needle
> til blood appears, in order to coax them to take hold. . . .
> Do not detach leeches forcibly, or else there may be violent haemor-
> rhage. . . .
> 1043. The use of leeches is beneficial in subcutaneous maladies like
> serpiginous ulcers, morphew, impetiginous ulcers, and the like (n.d., pp.
> 513–514].

During the seventeenth and eighteenth centuries into the early
years of the nineteenth century, the popularity of leeches as a means
of blood-letting prompted the publication of several reviews on the
subject, a well-known example being Johnson's A *Treatise on the
Medicinal Leech; Including its Medical and Natural History, with a
Description of its Anatomical Structure; also, Remarks upon the Diseases, Preservation and Management of Leeches* (1816). This enthusiasm reached mammoth proportions in France, possibly as a result
of the extraordinary influence of the French physician Francois Broussais (1772–1838). Broussais believed that all diseases were due to inflammation caused by irritation within the gastrointestinal tract. In
order to reduce this irritation, remedies consisting of diet and bleeding
were applied, frequently using leeches for the latter purpose. Indeed,

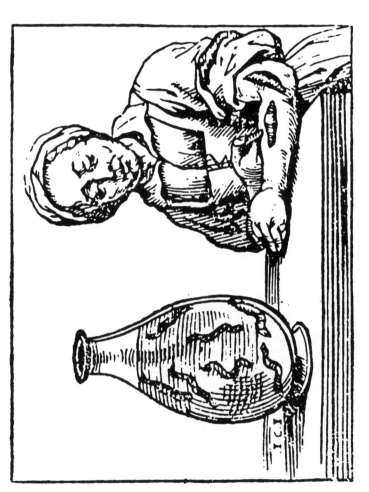

FIG. 16.1. A seventeenth-century woodcut by Guillelme Bossche, showing a woman seated at a table. A jar of leeches is on the table. She is applying a leech to her own forearm. *Source:* Bossche, G. (1639), *Historia Medica,* Brussels, p. 431. Courtesy of the National Library of Medicine, History of Medicine Division, Bethesda, MD.

Broussais was said to have had a standing order to apply thirty leeches to the skin of each of his patients almost as a matter of routine (Payton, 1981a). (The frequency of blood tests—some may call it blood-letting—in present-day hospitals is somewhat reminiscent of this practice.) Leech consumption in France increased to such an extent that the number of the worms imported to keep up with the demand increased from 100,000 in the year 1824 to 33,000,000 in 1827 (Sigerist, 1933, p. 289). The craze for leeches even extended to wearing clothes decorated with a leech motif. Following the death of Broussais, "leechmania," as this enthusiasm for leeches has sometimes been referred to (Rao, Bailie, and Bailey, 1985), rapidly faded away.

With the slow disappearance of their natural habitats as land was put to other uses, leeches became harder to find. A recent article, with the intriguing title of "The little suckers have made a comeback" (Conniff, 1987), mentioned the development of a commercial leech farm in Wales during the 1980s to replenish dwindling supplies of the parasite for both clinical and research purposes. Surgeons have returned to leeches in recent years in order to reduce the swelling and congestion of replants and skin flaps following reconstructive and plastic surgery (Rao et al., 1985). Others have applied leeches to remove blood from hematomas located around the eyes, particularly following trauma (Bunker, 1981).

Perhaps of greater importance in the renaissance of the leech than these few clinical uses has been a renewed scientific interest in the biologically active substances in leech saliva. It is well known that after a leech disengages itself from the skin, bleeding may continue for a prolonged period from the area of the bite. Indeed, this was considered such a problem that a surgical textbook of the nineteenth century by John Eric Erichsen gave detailed instructions to physicians on how to stop a hemorrhage from a leech-bite if it could not be controlled by ordinary means: "a piece of nitrate of silver scraped to a point, or a heated wire introduced into the bite, previously wiped dry, or a needle with a twisted suture over and around it, may be required" (1881, p. 151). Haycraft demonstrated that this excessive bleeding was due to an anticoagulant factor in leech saliva:

> The blood flowing from a leech-bite is not readily stopped, often flowing for upwards of an hour after the animal has been removed. The blood within the body of the creature remains fluid for an indefinite time; and when ejected

it is found to have lost its coagulability. These are facts known to every surgeon, but they have received no explanation.

While endeavouring to solve one very difficult problem, "why the blood does not coagulate within the living blood-vessels," the above facts came to my mind and promised to throw some light on the general question.

The explanation which at once suggested itself to me was, that probably the leech secretes some ferment-containing-juice which antagonises the blood ferment, preventing coagulation within its body, enough remaining around the edges of the wound to prevent for some time the outflowing blood from clotting; the blood remaining fluid, in fact, until the leech ferment is all washed away.

It will be seen that this explanation is in the main correct [1884, pp. 478–479].

One of the more interesting applications of the anticoagulant factor, named hirudin after the class Hirudinea, was mentioned by Abel, Rowntree, and Turner in early studies of an artificial kidney machine and dialysis at Johns Hopkins University:

As already stated, an extract obtained from the medicinal leech is employed in our method of vividiffusion to render the blood incoagulable. In consequence of the high price of hirudin, the anticoagulative principle of the leech, we now prepare for ourselves an active extract of this principle [1914, p. 302].

The authors not only described in detail how they prepared this leech extract but in an interesting aside also outlined the financial benefits obtained by making it themselves from leeches purchased in the United States rather than buying the commercial product or purchasing leeches from overseas:

Hirudin costs $27.50 a gram. We have used more than half a gram in a single experiment of long duration on a large dog. Good medicinal leeches from France can be bought in lots of one hundred or more from cupping barbers at the rate of $6.00 a hundred. Hynson, Westcott & Co., of Baltimore, inform us that they hope to be able to furnish the best leeches at $20 to $25 a thousand. As a single leech may yield 8 mgm. of active hirudin to extraction with water, the saving that results from making the extract is considerable [1914, p. 302].

In the years that followed, as drugs such as heparin and warfarin became available, hirudin saw limited clinical use as an anticoagulant. However, additional biologically and pharmacologically active substances were also isolated from leech saliva, including a spreading factor called hyaluronidase that enhances the absorption and dispersion of substances in tissues, a collagenase, a fibrinase that disrupts clots, and a material that prevents platelet aggregation (Lent, 1986). Whether

LES AMIS.

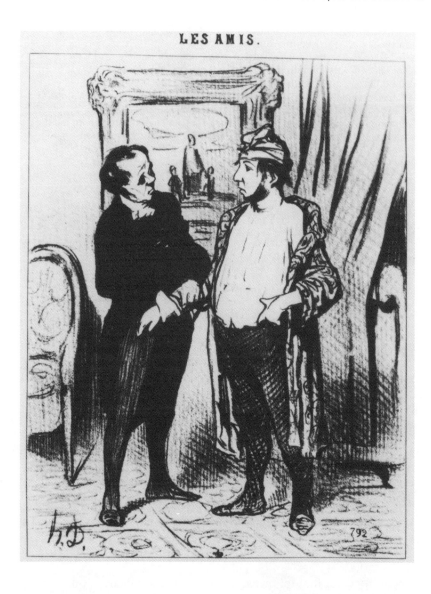

FIG. 16.2. A print by Honoré Daumier, the French caricaturist and artist, appearing in 1845, entitled "Les Amis," in which a physician tells a patient, as translated from the accompanying French caption: "I am going to apply thirty leeches to the epigastrium [the area over the stomach], and if tomorrow morning I do not find you stronger, I will reapply sixty!" *Source:* Courtesy of Yale Medical Historical Library, New Haven, CT.

these products will have clinical application remains to be seen. In addition extensive neuroanatomical and neurobiological studies of these creatures have been carried out, particularly in an attempt to understand their unusual feeding behavior (Payton, 1981b; Green and Gilby, 1983; Dickinson and Lent, 1984; Lent, 1985). For the moment, the leech not only perseveres but continues to be of interest.

The ubiquity of the leech in past centuries was not limited to the practice of medicine. Payton (1984) described some of the medical, biological, and popular illustrations of the medicinal leech that have appeared over the last eight hundred years, ranging from twelfth-century Chinese illustrations to lithographs by satirists during the height of the leech craze in France (Figure 16.2). A poem by William Wordsworth entitled "Resolution and Independence" not only portrayed the solitary life of a leech gatherer whose job it was to harvest leeches by wading barelegged in marshes, allowing his legs to serve as bait for the parasite, but in addition suggested the decreasing supply of the creatures in early nineteenth-century England:

> He told, that to these waters he had come
> To gather leeches, being old and poor:
> Employment hazardous and wearisome!
> And he had many hardships to endure:
> From pond to pond he roamed, from moor to moor;
> Housing, with God's good help, by choice or
>   chance;
> And in this way he gained an honest
>   maintenance. . . .
>
> He with a smile did then his words repeat;
> And said that, gathering leeches, far and wide
> He travelled; stirring thus about his feet
> The waters of the pools where they abide.
> "Once I could meet with them on every side;
> But they have dwindled long by slow decay;
> Yet still I persevere, and find them where I may."
>   [1807, pp. 196–197]

A print by the English artist George Walker during the early years of the nineteenth century depicted a similar method of harvesting leeches: women wading into pools in which leeches lived, waiting for the parasites to attach themselves, and then removing them quickly from their legs before the skin was broken (Einstein, 1978).

What the future holds for the leech in medicine is not possible to predict. A symbiotic relationship that has survived for over 2,000 years, however, is unlikely to disappear overnight, and indeed, the closing decades of the twentieth century have already seen a revival of interest in this amazing creature.

17

Music and Healing

Music has charms to soothe a savage breast,
To soften rocks, or bend a knotted oak.
[Congreve, 1697, p. 375]

No friend like music when the heart is broken,
To mend its wings and give it flight again.
[Hicky, n.d., p. 88]

THE ancient Greeks regarded Apollo as a god of both music and healing, leading Meinecke to comment that "Music and medicine therefore were intimately commingled in his [Apollo's] divine nature as an integrated unity" (1948, p. 48). Aesculapius (or Asclepius), recognized in Greek and Roman mythology as the son of Apollo, has traditionally been considered the patron of the healing arts, a fact acknowledged by all physicians who have taken the Hippocratic Oath on entering the medical profession—"I swear by Apollo the physician, and Aesculapius . . . and all the gods and goddesses" (Hippocrates, c. 400 B.C.b, p. 779). The medical skills of Asclepius were further described in the following citation from ancient Greek writings, as quoted by Edelstein:

those whosoever came suffering from the sores of nature, or with their limbs wounded . . . he loosed and delivered divers of them from diverse pains, tending some of them with kindly songs, giving to others a soothing potion, or,

125

haply, swathing their limbs with simples, or restoring others by the knife [1937, p. 224].

A well-known passage from I Samuel 16:23 in the *Old Testament* suggests that the healing or soothing effect of music was used in biblical times for treating what may have been a psychological or emotional problem: "And whenever the evil spirit from God was upon Saul, David took the lyre and played it with his hand; so Saul was refreshed, and was well, and the evil spirit departed from him."

Further descriptions of the healing power of music as applied by the ancients 2,000 years ago are found in the writings of Aulus Gellius, a Roman author of the second century:

> I [Aulus Gellius] ran across the statement very recently in the book of Theophrastus [entitled] On Inspiration that many men have believed and put their belief on record, that when gouty pains in the hips are most severe they are relieved if a flute-player plays soothing measures. That snake-bites are cured by the music of the flute, when played skillfully and melodiously, is also stated in a book of Democritus, entitled On Deadly Infections, in which he shows that the music of the flute is medicine for many ills that flesh is heir to. So very close is the connection between the bodies and the minds of men, and therefore between physical and mental ailments and their remedies [Edelstein, 1937, pp. 234–235].

The ancient Greeks recognized different forms of music according to its influence upon the body:

> The Dorian influences to modesty and purity; the Phrygian stimulates to fierce combat; the Aeolian composes mental disturbances and induces sleep; the Ionian whets dull intellects and kindles a desire for heavenly things; the Lydian soothes the soul when oppressed with excessive cares [Meinecke, 1948, p. 69].

Thus Greek and Roman physicians prescribed music appropriate to the problem being treated—Asclepiades "treated insanity through the medium of harmonious sounds" (Meinecke, 1948, p. 75), Celsus "recommends music, cymbals, and sounds to dispel the melancholy thoughts symptomatic of certain types of mental derangement" (p. 75), Caelius Aurelianus "includes the music of the double-flute in the Phrygian key, recommended for such as are dejected at one time, and in a rage at another, since it is both pleasing and stimulating (p. 75), while "Cato has preserved an incantation for the cure of sprains, and Varro another for that of gout" (p. 83).

Many years later, reports appeared describing the association of music with a strange sickness called *tarantism*, present in Italy for several hundred years before finally disappearing during the eighteenth century (Sigerist, 1943). The disease was thought to afflict those bitten by the tarantula, a spider that some believed was poisonous. Symptoms recurred periodically, particularly during the hot summer months, when the presumed poisonous effects of the spider were mysteriously activated. On these occasions, groups of patients gathered together and danced in great excitement to the sound of special musical pieces called tarantellas, often indulging at the same time in excesses of behavior such as whipping each other or performing indecent acts. This music, played by roving bands of musicians, was, in the opinion of the public, said to be the only effective remedy for this disorder. In a report entitled A *Dissertation of the Anatomy, Bitings and other Effects of the venemous Spider, call'd Tarantula*, the author, a seventeenth-century physician called Giorgio Baglivi, explained how the music prompted violent dancing, the beneficial effects of which occurred through the following mechanism:

> It being manifest . . . that music ravishes healthy persons into such actions as imitate the harmony they hear, we easily adjust our opinion of the effects of music in the cure of persons stung by a tarantula. It is probable, that the very swift motion impressed upon the air by musical instruments, and communicated by the air to the skin, and so to the spirits and blood, does, in some measure, dissolve and dispel their growing coagulation; and that the effects of the dissolution increase as the sound itself increases, till, at last, the humors retrieve their primitive fluid state, by virtue of these repeated shakings and vibrations; upon which the patient revives gradually, moves his limbs, gets upon his legs, groans, jumps about with violence, till the sweat breaks and carries off the seeds of the poison [Sigerist, 1943, pp. 223–224].

In reviewing this unusual sickness, in which music and the resultant dancing were apparently relevant to the cure, the noted medical historian Henry Sigerist suggested that rather than being caused by the bite of the tarantula, the disease was a nervous disorder peculiar to the region in which it occurred, possibly manifesting itself in certain ancient pagan and orgiastic rites which "appeared as symptoms of a disease" (1943, p. 226). Although such an explanation is speculative, the disease and its treatment once again demonstrate an interesting and unusual relationship, whether real or perceived, between medicine and the healing power of music.

Closer to our own time, Canon Harford, in a letter to the editor of the *Lancet*, asked the question "Whether soft low music might not be used with advantage as a curative assistant in a considerable number of cases of illness, more particularly those in which the nerves are specially concerned?" (1891, p. 43). The author outlined a plan to organize performing artists for this purpose, adding a note in his correspondence that "Miss Florence Nightingale has expressed her full concurrence with the objects of the Mission of St. Cecilia [the supporters of this project], and wishes it God-Speed" (1891, p. 44). The following year, Hunter wrote that music played at his infirmary helped diminish pain in many patients, in addition to which "seven out of ten noted cases were benefited in so far as a reduction of temperature was recorded" (1892, p. 923).

In the late nineteenth century and early years of the twentieth century, several studies were performed in order to examine the physiological functions of the body that might be affected by music. Davison referred to earlier work of Dogiel in which it was demonstrated that music might cause either a rise or fall in blood pressure depending upon the pitch, loudness, and tone color of the sound, and that "in the variations of the blood-pressure the idiosyncrasies of the individual, whether man or animal, are plainly apparent, and even the nationality, in the case of man, has some effect" (1899, p. 1160).

Hyde evaluated the effects of different types of musical selections upon the cardiovascular system, i.e., on blood pressure, pulse rate, electrocardiogram, "in individuals who are known to be fond of music, [and] persons indifferent or not sensitive to music" (1924, p. 213). Three contrasting musical pieces were played—"First the record of the Boston Symphony Orchestra of Tschaickowsky's Tragic Symphony characterized by slow minor movements. Second, the Toreador's brilliant description of the bull fight, from Carmen . . . and third the National Emblem, a stirring rhythmical march by Sousa's Band" (1924, p. 215). In noting that differences in response to these selections were related not only to the type of music being played but also to the musical background of the subject being tested, Hyde concluded that "with this method the proper sort of music may be prescribed and thus a scientific employment of the power inherent in music may prove a valuable adjunct to psychotherapy in the treatment of convalescent or other patients sensitive to music" (1924, p. 222).

Hyde referred to one particular patient with "an extreme auricular acceleration, or auricular flutter" (1924, p. 221) in whom this irregularity decreased or ceased when the soothing music of a lullaby was played. Indeed, the objective data Hyde obtained appeared to add credence to the previously mentioned beliefs of the ancient Greeks in the use of musical forms to produce specific effects upon the body, e.g., Dorian, Phrygian, Aeolian, and others. Additional studies by Vincent and Thompson substantiated the observation that the blood pressures of subjects grouped into musical, moderately musical, and non-musical sets responded "differently in relation to variations of volume, melody, rhythm, pitch, and type of music" (1929, p. 537).

Many of the early reports on the psychological effects of music therapy were anecdotal or descriptive in style, often referring to well-known individuals who benefited from this form of treatment (Cook, 1981). One of the first major attempts at evaluating the psychological influence of music in a large number of patients was described during the late nineteenth century by Dr. Sebastian Wimmer, a somewhat homey approach to scientific investigation when compared with the stringent requirements of present-day research protocols:

> In 1878 some very curious and interesting experiments were carried on in New York city [sic], at the Randall's Island Asylum. Fourteen hundred females (insane) were congregated in the large entertainment hall of the institution and subjected to a strain of piano music for half an hour, when the general effects were noted as follows: the pulse was raised, the patients became restless, and there was a marked desire to keep time with the music. They were all susceptible to the rhythm, and its effect was decidedly stimulating. Melody without any very decided or certain tempo was without effect excepting in those cases where the force of association was still active. In a case of chronic melancholia the playing of "Home, Sweet Home" invariably brought the patient to her knees, where she began to recite the Lord's Prayer in an apparent ecstasy of devotion. In another case—one of acute mania—the patient's pulse was elevated from 78 to 106 beats, the patient not showing any other signs of excitation save the involuntary twitching of the facial muscles. Cantabile music seemed to have an effect, in the worst cases, similar to that which it exercises upon certain animals, the person being disposed to lie down and go to sleep under its influence. The results of all these experiments were markedly beneficial, and, by frequent repetitions, many of the patients showed great improvement. The effects, in almost every instance, of the pronounced rhythm were involuntary, the movements of the limbs and facial muscles being attributed to reflex action. It seems plausible to me that music can exert a wonderful influence over an individual whose nervous system has been shattered in any way by gradually soothing that system and bringing it into harmonious accord with the spirit of the composition interpreted [Wimmer, 1889, p. 259].

Several years later, Shoemaker, in referring to the use of distinct musical forms for different conditions—reminiscent once more of the ancient Greeks—stated that "music, of a kind suited to the actual condition of the patient, may be a potent factor in restoration, through its special influence upon the nervous system" (1901, p. 292), concluding that "[w]e must learn how to adapt the character of harmonious notes to the requirements of the system" (1901, p. 294). Notwithstanding such comments, however, a certain degree of reservation about the uniqueness of music therapy in treating psychological disorders was expressed by Edwards in a letter to the editor of *American Medicine*, indicating that "music has the same effect upon insane as upon sane people, certainly no special curative influence" (1905, p. 305).

In more recent years, at times in spite of the paucity of "hard" data, there has been sufficient interest, enthusiasm, and support to warrant the use of music for a variety of different purposes, both medical and nonmedical, in an effort to obtain its apparent psychological and physiological benefits. For example, music has been shown to increase efficiency of production in industrial plants (Cardinell, 1948), to be beneficial in the care of psychiatric patients (Altshuler and Shebesta, 1941), to enhance the quality of life while palliative care is being provided to patients with advanced malignant disease (Munro and Mount, 1978), to assist in the management of the developmentally disabled (Boxill, 1985), and to improve the physical and psychological well-being of the elderly in long-term care institutions (Mason, 1978). Indeed, a recent plea was made for nurses to consider this form of therapy more than they have in the past, stating that "music appears to have a wide variety of applications in the patient care setting. If fully appreciated and used judiciously, music has the potential of becoming a valuable nursing intervention toward the achievement of comprehensive patient care" (Cook, 1981, p. 264).

It is tempting to speculate that the cardiorespiratory effects of music might also be of benefit when used in conjunction with standard forms of therapy for managing patients with heart and lung ailments, particularly in treating cardiac arrhythmias, in restoring normal hemodynamic function, and in reducing pain and apprehension. If such benefits can be demonstrated for these and other medical problems, there may well be a revised interest in the triple therapeutic approach suggested long ago according to the myths of ancient Greece: "Asclepius treated sick people with drugs, with the knife and with soothing songs" (Sigerist, 1943, p. 212).

18

The Medical Uses of Wine
Throughout the Ages

Good wine is a good familiar creature if it be well
used.
　　[Shakespeare—*Othello*, Act II, Scene iii, Line 315]

A clay tablet inscribed in Sumerian cuneiform script over 4,000
years ago records one of the earliest known references to a wine-
containing medical prescription—a powder infused with "kushumma"
wine (Kramer, 1954, p. 78). According to Leake, wine was administered as a vehicle in 12 of 260 prescriptions identified in the Hearst
Medical Papyrus of ancient Egypt dating back to 1550 B.C. (1952, p.
73). Additional recipes or formulas specifying wine as an ingredient
are recorded in the famous Ebers Medical Papyrus of the same period
for use in a wide variety of medical problems (Ebbell, 1937). The ro
(mouthful) referred to in the following prescriptions from this papyrus
was an Egyptian measure equal to 15 milliliters or one tablespoon.

> Remedy for dejection: colocynth 4 ro, honey 4 ro, are mixed together,
> eaten and swallowed with beer 10 ro or wine 5 ro [1937, p. 30].
> Another [remedy] to cause purgation: 6 senna (pods) (which are like beans
> from Crete) and fruit . . . (which is called colocynth) are ground fine, put on
> honey and eaten by the man and swallowed with sweet wine 5 ro [1937, p.
> 32].
> Another [remedy to cause the stomach to receive bread]: fat flesh 2 ro,

wine 5 ro, raisin 2 ro, figs 2 ro, celery 2 ro, sweet beer 25 ro, are boiled,
strained and taken for 4 days [1937, p. 63].

    Another [remedy to expel epilepsy in a man]: testicles of an ? ass, are
ground fine, put in wine and drunk by the man; it (i.e. the epilepsy) will cease
immediately [1937, p. 105].

In all likelihood, wine served as a tranquilizer and sedative during
biblical times, as these lines from Proverbs 31:6 in the *Old Testament*
suggest:

> Give strong drink to him who is perishing,
>   and wine to those in bitter distress;
> let them drink and forget their poverty,
>   and remember their misery no more.

In addition, the Babylonian Talmud, a collection of Hebrew civil
and religious laws said to have been compiled about fourteen to fifteen
hundred years ago, acknowledged the use of wine both as a medicine—"At the head of all medicine am I, Wine; only when there is
no wine are drugs required" (Babylonian Talmud, n.d.a, p. 235)—and
as a substance with nutritional value—"It [wine] sustains and makes
glad, whereas bread sustains but does not cheer" (Babylonian Talmud,
n.d.b, p. 223). Further recognition of wine's medical beneficence can
also be found in the *New Testament*, 1 Timothy 5:23: "No longer
drink only water, but use a little wine for the sake of your stomach
and your frequent ailments."

    Yet a further medical use of wine in ancient times is commented
upon in an ancient Sanskrit medical text, as excerpted by Lucia:
" . . . the patient should be given to eat what he wishes and wine to
drink before the operation, so that he may not faint and may not feel
the knife" (1963a, p. 28). Film buffs may appreciate a parallel between
the removal of an arrow or bullet from the protagonist of a cowboy
or gangster movie, aided by the liberal use of a bottle of whiskey, and
this ancient Hindu practice of employing wine as an anesthetic agent.

    Wine was utilized by the ancient Greeks for dressing wounds, for
fevers, for increasing the urine flow, and for treating gastrointestinal
symptoms, with different wines having distinctive effects, as noted by
Hippocrates in *On Regimen in Acute Diseases*:

Wherefore the sweet [wine] affects the head less than the strong, attacks the brain less, evacuates the bowels more than the other, but induces swelling of the spleen and liver; it does not agree with bilious persons, for it causes them to thirst. . . . [I]t in general is less diuretic than wine which is strong and thin; but sweet wine is more expectorant than the other [c. 400. B.C. a, pp. 298–299].

In his *Aphorisms*, Hippocrates added: "Drinking strong wine cures hunger" [c. 400. B.C.b, p. 708]. Thus, advantage was taken of the diverse characteristics of the various wines in prescribing for specific medical conditions. Dioscorides similarly discussed wines in great detail, again distinguishing particular medical uses of specific wines:

But generally all unmixed & simple wine, hard by nature, is warming, easily digested, good for ye stomach, wetting ye appetite, nourishing, soporiferous, inducing a good colour. . . . And it is effectual for ye windiness of long continuance, & ye gnawing of ye Hypochondrium, and ye distension & singultus stomachi, & for ye flux of ye entrails, and of ye belly, & it is good for sweaters & such as faint thereby, but especially ye white & old & sweet-smelling wines; but the old & sweet are more convenient both for ye griefs about ye bladder & kidnies, as also for wounds & inflammations [c. 70 A.D., pp. 605–606].

About 100 years later, Galen (131–201 A.D.) observed that the wounds of gladiators treated with dressings soaked with red wine did not become putrid. He commented, according to Lucia, that "I am in the habit of cleaning the sinus [of fistulous abscesses] with wine alone, sometimes with honeyed wine. . . . This wine should be neither sweet nor astringent" (1963a, p. 71). Thus the antiseptic benefits of wine were recognized.

Avicenna, during the great era of Arabian medicine, discussed the effects of wine on the pulse and on body temperature (n.d., pp. 313–314) and on digestive functions (n.d., p. 410). In addition, he also described remedies to neutralize the harmful actions of wine:

805. If wine has an injurious effect on the body and is heating to the liver, the diet should include some dish containing for instance the juice of (sour) unripe grapes, and the like . . . such as pomegranate, and tart things like citron.

If the wine is liable to go to the head, one should take less and take it dilute and clarified. After the meal, he should take such as quince with his wine.

If the harmful effect of wine consists in being heating to the stomach, the dessert should include toasted myrtle-seeds; and one should suck a few camphor lozenges and other astringent and acrid things.

806. As you know, old wine is like a medicine [n.d., pp. 410–411].

Arnald (or Arnold) of Villanova (c. 1235–1311), a well-known and colorful medical personage of the Middle Ages, wrote a popular and influential book on the medicinal uses of wines entitled *Liber de vinis*. In an extract from this book, quoted by Lucia, Arnald indicated that raisin wine, to which cinnamon was added,

> is a wine that is proper for sick old people, also for melancholics and phleg-matics, and it particularly makes women fat. It eases the chest, strengthens the stomach, adds substance to the liver and strengthens it. It warms the blood, opposes putrefaction, and removes nausea and mucosity of the stomach. It is also useful for coughing and asthma, and it naturally loosens the hardened bowels and astringes the loose bowels, such as in dysentery and similar conditions. It has the faculty of strengthening the retentive and expulsive function. It is good for short breath and for the cardiac disease [Lucia, 1963a, p. 105].

The potential benefits of wine for such a multiplicity of ailments no doubt added much to the appeal of this book.

During this same period of the thirteenth century, Aldobrandino da Siena wrote *Li livres dou santé*, a practical manual of health that was said to be the first medical book composed in French rather than in classic Latin. In discussing the section devoted to diet in this work, Jones commented:

> Aldobrandino recommends wines which are neither too new nor too old, and his overall verdict is that wine, taken in moderation, fortifies the natural heat of the body, nourishes, makes man joyous, aids nature in its course, and delays the onset of old age [1984, pp. 135–136].

The blandishments offered by the aforementioned texts are highly reminiscent of similar inducements found in the numerous publications currently available on health, exercise, and diet. Indeed, what would the pharmaceutical industry not give to develop all these medicinal attributes of wine into a remedy that would pass muster by the United States Food and Drug Administration!

A French army surgeon of the Renaissance, Ambroise Paré (1510–1590), found that wounds could be treated successfully with dressings containing wine or other forms of alcohol. In addition, according to Lucia in quoting from one of Paré's works, " . . . I [Paré] made him [a patient] drinke wine moderately tempered with water, knowing that it restores and quickens the vital forces" (1963a, p. 118). Further observations on the medical uses of wine extended to the treatment of heart diseases, with the English physician William Heberden stating in his masterful work on angina pectoris that "Wine, and spirituous liquors, and opium, afford considerable relief" (1802, p. 367).

Textbooks of materia medica and therapeutics written during the last half of the nineteenth century described wine in great detail, Vinum Portense (port wine) and Vinum Xericum (sherry wine) being officially recognized by the United States Pharmacopoeia (Bartholow, 1882, p. 392). Biddle noted that "Port contains tannic acid, and is preferred in dysentery, diarrhoea, etc., for its astringency" (1880, p. 200), while Bartholow listed dyspepsia, diarrhoea, chlorosis, the recovery period after an acute sickness, and various acute diseases and inflammations, as some of the conditions in which wine could be used with benefit. He added:

> Next to their use in fevers, wines are most frequently prescribed, and with the greatest advantage, in *surgical practice*, for the *consequences of wounds* and *injuries*, to *support the powers of life under protracted and profuse suppuration*, and to favor digestion and assimilation in the course of convalescence from surgical diseases [Bartholow, 1882, p. 396].

In an address before members of the British Medical Association during the early years of the twentieth century, James Macdonald summarized the medical profession's attitude as it then existed toward the therapeutic role of alcohol: "Alcohol is a drug, and as such must be administered with the same precision and discrimination which we employ in prescribing other powerful drugs. Given with these precautions, alcohol is an invaluable remedy in the treatment of disease" (1909, p. 268). Thus, during the first half of the current century, wine was recommended in clinical practice not only for its sedative action (Clendening, 1935, p. 76) but also for its nutritional benefits in treating the cachexia of chronic diseases: "A tuberculous youth, with appetite gone, losing weight, sick of the sight of food, may have his nutrition improved almost beyond belief by the use of sherry wine with his meals" (1935, p. 145).

Numerous publications have focused upon the benefits of alcohol in cardiovascular and emotional disorders. In 1928, Harlow Brooks discussed the use of alcohol for the circulatory defects of old age, commenting that "brandy, whiskey, or the heavy wines, as port, sherry, and the like, are the preferable forms to use [for angina pectoris]" (1928, p. 200), while wines as well as other alcoholic beverages could be used with benefit in "hypertension with its attendant apprehension, melancholy and general discomfort" (p. 201). Within this context, Brooks also made reference to the well-known aphorism attributed to Osler "that alcohol is the milk of old age" (p. 200).

By measuring a rise in skin temperature, a vasodilating effect of alcohol on the affected limbs of patients with peripheral circulatory disorders was demonstrated by Cook and Brown, who concluded: "Alcohol gives many of these patients great relief; it occasionally helps to tide them over episodes of pain, and amputation frequently can be obviated or delayed" (1932, p. 452). Palarea reviewed in detail the physiologic effects of alcohol upon the body in various medical and surgical disciplines, summarizing his findings as follows:

> When administered properly, ethanol is a safe, inexpensive and effective drug. In the management of certain disorders it can be of value as a sedative, analgesic, autonomic stimulant, high-calorie food, poison antidote, cooler, solvent, antiseptic, rubefacient, vasodilator, diagnostic agent, defoaming agent or diuretic [1963, p. 942].

In an attempt to evaluate emotional stress objectively, Greenberg and Carpenter performed an interesting experiment in which "the basic skin conductance . . . has been taken as a quantitative measure of the level of emotional tension—an 'emotional tension index'—associated with sustained performance of a standardized task" (1957, p. 198). On administering wine or other forms of alcohol while making the above measurements, these investigators observed that "[a]mounts of alcoholic beverage considerably less than those commonly observed to cause intoxicated behavior have been shown to reduce emotional tension, as measured by skin conductance, to a significant degree" (1957, p. 203).

Research has continued in more recent years, attempting to answer many of the questions and doubts that still exist regarding the benefits that may be obtained from the therapeutic use of alcohol. A study by Turner, Bennett, and Hernandez from the Johns Hopkins Medical Institutions, after reviewing the published data and defining the limits of moderate alcoholic intake, indicated that such use by adults "may reduce the risk of myocardial infarction, improve the quality of life of the elderly, relieve stress, and contribute to nutrition" (1981, p. 53).

In the conclusion to his book *A History of Wine as Therapy*,

Lucia wrote, "To the medical historian, it is of particular interest that science has now corroborated a great deal of the empirical evidence amassed during the four thousand years of the illustrious history of the oldest of medicines—wine" (1963a, p. 208). In spite of such statements, however, wine is generally no longer listed in pharmacopoeias and formularies, although a tonic consisting of beef, iron, and wine was still officially mentioned during the mid-1940s in the twenty-fourth edition of *The Dispensatory of the United States of America* (Osol and Farrar, 1947, pp. 132–133). In part this might be due to the anti-alcohol crusades of recent years; in part it may be that the various benefits ascribed to wine and other alcoholic beverages can now be obtained from more specific and potent pharmacologic agents. It does seem, however, that by not taking advantage of a therapy that may "give comfort and soothe the last lap of life's troublous transit" (Rolleston, 1924, p. 215), that may provide "Balm for the autumnal years" (Lucia, 1963b, p. 170), and that, unlike other medical treatments, may also give a certain degree of pleasure to an ailing patient without causing distressing side effects, something has been lost, if not in the science then perhaps in the art of medicine.

Section III

On the Road to Contemporary Cardiac Care

INCLUDED in this section are discussions of how several medical therapies, surgical interventions, and technologic procedures evolved into treatments and practices that are now part of contemporary cardiac care.

Exercise was a traditional and well-established part of medical therapeutics for many years prior to attaining its present level of usage in physical therapy departments and in cardiovascular evaluation and exercise programs. Indeed, recommendations for exercise from the eighteenth and nineteenth centuries could well be inserted into modern textbooks with few changes needed to make them current.

Anticoagulants as they developed from knowledge of a disease of cattle and from a rat poison; rauwolfia, the forerunner of modern drugs used in the treatment of hypertension and a therapy that had many applications in ancient Hindu medicine; nitroglycerine and related compounds that developed from the interesting observations of physicians during the nineteenth century, medications that no respectable present-day physician would be without in treating cardiac patients; quinidine, an anti-arrhythmic drug, derived from a preparation found in the bark of a tree that was used for the treatment of malaria; and recently available beta blockers, the new boy on the block, with a fascinating history of pharmacologic investigation reaching back to the early years of the twentieth century: these are some of the medications that have been of value in contemporary cardiology and have in some instances prepared the way for other drugs with similar properties.

Also discussed in this section are heart surgery and the technologic achievements, such as those related to the heart-lung machine, cardiac catheterization, and the field of anesthesiology, that made such surgery possible. Cardiac pacing became available as electrophysiological research, with roots extending back to observations made two hundred or more years ago, matured, and as opportunities became available through progress in pacemaker technology. Heart valve surgery hinged upon a detailed understanding of valve function and cardiac hemodynamics, and upon the discovery of suitable materials that could be inserted into the body to withstand the wear and tear of constant use. The startling and awesome achievement of heart transplantation during the 1960s, dependent as it was on knowledge gained from many years of research in the laboratory and on information contributed by many medical disciplines, has moved from the realm of fantasy to become a reality.

And finally, the recent appearance of echocardiography is reviewed. This procedure, the origins of which can be traced to the development of ultrasound and of reflected wave forms in other scientific disciplines and in industry, has made a significant impact upon the present-day practice of cardiology, with promises of more to come.

19

Exercise and Health: From British Prisons to Cardiac Rehabilitation Programs

Reading is to the mind, what exercise is to the body.
[Addison and Steele, 1709–1710]

A NCIENT Chinese and Indian medical writings contain numerous statements about exercise in restoring and in maintaining health. Licht (1965) noted that the *Ayer-Veda*, an anatomy book of ancient India, advised exercise and massage for chronic rheumatism. Ganorkar and Mandal wrote that Shushruta, the great Indian surgeon of this ancient period,

> recommended the daily practice of exercise. While commenting on its values he [Shushruta] further states that exercise makes the body stout and strong, helps the symmetrical growth of muscles and limbs, improves the complexion, and the digestive function power, prevents laziness and makes the body light, glossy and compact. . . . It leads to freedom from disease and is the best means of reducing corpulency [1973, pp. 134–135].

In the *Huan Ti Nei Ching Su Wên—The Yellow Emperor's Classic of Internal Medicine,* the great work of ancient Chinese medicine that may have been written over 4,000 years ago, the Yellow Emperor engages in a dialogue with his minister Ch'i Po about a variety of medical topics. As translated by Veith, the benefits of exercise are

141

referred to in the course of their discussions: "After a night of sleep people should get up early (in the morning); they should walk briskly around the yard; they should loosen their hair and slow down their movements (body); by these means they can (fulfill) their wish to live healthfully" (Veith, 1949, p. 102). Elsewhere in the same text, the comment is made that "These diseases [paralysis, chills and fever] are most fittingly treated with breathing exercises, massage of skin and flesh, and exercises of hands and feet" (1949, p. 148).

Turning to Western civilization, one of the earliest Greek physicians to write about therapeutic exercises was Herodicus, born about 480 B.C. His enthusiastic prescriptions were at times considered excessive, with one of his students, Hippocrates, quoted as saying, "He [Herodicus] killed the febrile with walking, too much wrestling and fomentation. There is nothing more pernicious for the febrile than wrestling, walking and massage. It is like treating a disturbance with a disturbance" (Licht, 1965, p. 428).

In spite of this statement, numerous references to exercise in health and disease may be found throughout the works of Hippocrates (460–370 B.C.), with the following excerpt from *On the Articulations* demonstrating a clear understanding of the benefits to be derived from physical therapy: "In a word, all parts of the body which were made for active use, if moderately used and exercised at the labour to which they are habituated, become healthy, increase in bulk, and bear their age well, but when not used, and when left without exercise, they become diseased, their growth is arrested, and they soon become old" (Hippocrates, c. 400 B.C.b, p. 629).

Several other ancient Greek and Roman physicians also commented about exercise. One of these was Galen, expressing a careful approach in his book *On Hygiene*: "The attention should be closely applied to the exercising body, and it [the exercise] should be stopped at once when any adverse signs appear" (Licht, 1965, p. 431). Also cited by Licht is this strikingly modern principle stated by Caelius Aurelianus about postoperative exercises: "For the little additional motion cannot cause the wound to open again; on the contrary, it will aid in building up the patient's strength during the period of recovery" (p. 433).

Hieronymus Mercurialis (1530–1606), a professor at Padua, published a treatise on diseases of the skin and one of the early works on diseases of children. He is particularly remembered, however, for an important book on therapeutic exercises, *De Arte Gymnastica*, published in 1569. According to Licht, Mercurialis recommended that:

> (3) Exercises should be suited to each part of the body. (4) All healthy people should take exercise regularly. (5) Sick people should not be given exercises which might exacerbate existing conditions. (6) Special exercises should be prescribed for convalescent patients on an individual basis. (7) Persons who lead a sedentary life urgently need exercise [1965, pp. 437–438].

At the age of 33, Joseph-Clément Tissot (1747–1826) published his well-known *Gymnastique Médicinale et Chirurgicale*, outlining many important principles that continue to be relevant in present-day rehabilitation medicine:

> If, for example, after the healing of wounds, fistulae, whitlow, sprains, etc., there remains a difficulty in moving the joints, or if the joint difficulty depends on the stiffness and torpor of the extensors and flexors, it is up to the surgeon to select those exercises which are best indicated to restore motion [Tissot, 1780, p. 30].
>
> Is it necessary to give examples to prove that the abuse of rest is more dangerous than that of movement? At all times, right under our eyes, we see patients who have been forced to remain in bed for a long time. They usually leave the bed with crippled or ankylosed limbs; or they have developed a primary scurvy, or their convalescence is in itself a new disease. . . . Even the strongest horse, if allowed to remain inactive too long in the stable, loses his strength and vivacity. If a prolonged rest produces such a bad effect on the hard and elastic fibers of this animal, what must it do to the more sensitive fibers of men which are weaker and on those of women which are still more delicate? [p. 52].
>
> When the weight of the entire body presses against the side on which the patient lies, there frequently occur complications to the parts where the bones are prominent especially at the coccyx; the pressure which these parts experience is soon followed by inflammation and gangrene, if we are not watchful. . . .
>
> The remedy for all these complications . . . is to change the position of the patient often . . . [p. 80].
>
> Without going into the details of the causes and diagnosis [of apoplexy] . . . let us concern ourselves only with observing that the important point in its treatment consists in reawakening the reduced elasticity of the brain which involves the rest of the body, and by placing in action all those things which maintain watchfulness. Movement is capable of aiding these urgent indications. . . .
>
> Apoplectics must not remain in bed. . . .
>
> Once consciousness has returned, the patient must have motion; he will at first walk supported by assistants, and later he will get into a carriage or on a horse as his strength will permit [pp. 96–97].

That these views on various aspects of exercise, whose spirit and content are modern, were written over two centuries ago attests to the unusual talent and ability of their author.

The unique contribution of another Frenchman, Philippe Pinel, in bringing exercise and physical activity to the setting of psychiatric disorders should not be overlooked. In a chapter entitled "Varieties of bodily exercises including laborious occupations recommended for convalescents" in his well-known work A *Treatise on Insanity*, Pinel outlined the benefits of a work program, a combination of both physical and occupational therapy, for "convalescent maniacs" (1806, p. 193), noting:

> The whole day is thus occupied in salutary and refreshing exercises, which are interrupted only by short intervals of rest and relaxation. The fatigues of the day prepare the labourers for sleep and repose during the night. Hence it happens, that those whose condition does not place them above the necessity of submission to toil and labour, are almost always cured; whilst the grandee, who would think himself degraded by any exercises of this description, is generally incurable [1806, p. 195].

One of the earliest references to exercise for patients with cardiovascular diseases was written by William Stokes, the Irish physician perhaps better remembered for his eponymous associations with Adams-Stokes syndrome and Cheyne-Stokes respiration. In his book, *The Diseases of the Heart and the Aorta*, Stokes commented:

> In the present state of our knowledge, the adoption of the following principles in the management of a case of incipient fatty disease [fatty degeneration of the heart] seems justifiable:—
> 1. We must train the patient gradually but steadily to the giving up of all luxurious habits. He must adopt early hours, and pursue a system of graduated muscular exercise; and it will often happen that after perseverance in this system the patient will be enabled to take an amount of exercise with pleasure and advantage, which at first was totally impossible, owing to the difficulty of breathing which followed exertion. This treatment by muscular exercise is obviously more proper in younger persons than in those advanced in life. The symptoms of debility of the heart are often removable by a regulated course of gymnastics, or by pedestrian exercise, even in mountainous countries such as Switzerland, or the highlands of Scotland or Ireland. We may often observe in such persons the occurrence of what is commonly known as "getting the second wind," that is to say, during the first period of the day the patient suffers from dyspnoea and palpitations to an extreme degree, but by persevering, without overexertion, or after a short rest, he can finish his day's work, and even ascend high mountains with facility [1854, p. 357].

Strangely enough, a quantitative approach to diagnostic and therapeutic uses of exercise in managing cardiovascular diseases has been traced to the British prison system during the first half of the nineteenth century. William Cubitt, a civil engineer, was asked by prison officials to design a device that would provide activity for prisoners sentenced to hard labor. He responded by constructing a machine, "Variously termed a treadmill, treadwheel, everlasting staircase, and discipline mill" (Chapman, 1967, p. 7), on which prisoners could walk and exercise together for prolonged periods (Figure 19.1). However, reformers were critical of this invention, charging, as noted in another reference cited by Chapman, "that the Tread-wheel is, in reality, a species of torture, intruding itself under the semblance of labour" (p. 9).

At about the time when this machine was beginning to fall into disfavor, Dr. Edward Smith, a physician, physiologist, and a reformer himself, realized that the treadmill or treadwheel might be a useful instrument in his research. Smith performed experiments on prisoners working these machines at Coldbath-fields prison in London. From those studies he was able to obtain quantitative exercise data on respiratory rate, ventilatory volume, and pulse rate (Smith, 1857). Following this unusual beginning, procedures have evolved and been refined for quantifying and evaluating cardiac and respiratory performance during exercise. In recent years, the standard two-step exercise tolerance test of Master and Oppenheimer (1929) and the resurrected treadmill itself (Bruce, 1956) have been brought into diagnostic and research laboratories, a far cry from their use as instruments for providing hard labor for convicts in British jails over a hundred years ago.

Since the 1950s, many efforts have been made to better understand the relationship between coronary artery disease and physical activity. A significant publication on this subject by Morris and Crawford in England stated:

> Evidence has now been produced relating several aspects of clinical and subclinical coronary heart disease to physical activity of work. The general *hypothesis* may therefore be restated in *causal* terms that *physical activity of work is a protection against coronary (ischaemic) heart disease. Men in physically active jobs have less coronary heart disease during middle-age, what disease they have is less severe, and they develop it later than men in physically inactive jobs.* Since there are suggestions of other connexions between physical activity of work and cardiovascular disease of middle-age, and multiplying evidence from laboratory experiment of the beneficial effects of exercise on relevant cardiovascular physiology and pathology, the *speculation* may be advanced that

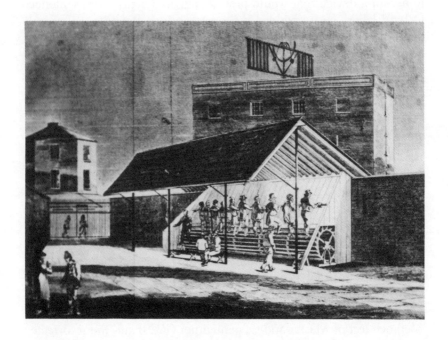

FIG. 19.1. An engraving showing prisoners at work on the treadwheels of a discipline mill at the House of Correction at Brixton, in Surrey, England. By continually climbing the steps that turned this wheel, the prisoners supplied power to operate machinery located in the millhouse behind the treadwheel for the purpose of grinding corn. Such a device provided Edward Smith with the opportunity to perform quantitative physiologic exercise studies (Chapman, 1967). *Source:* Proceedings of Public Societies: Society for the Improvement of Prison Discipline (with an engraving) (1823), Monthly Magazine, 56, No. 56:55–60. Engraving reproduced by permission of the editor of the *Journal of the History of Medicine and Allied Sciences* from Figure 7 in Chapman, C. B. (1967), Edward Smith (?1818–1874), physiologist, human ecologist, reformer. *J. Hist. Med. Allied Sci.*, 22:1–26.

habitual physical activity is a general factor of cardiovascular health in middle-age, and that coronary heart disease is in some respects a deprivation syndrome, a deficiency disease [1958, p. 1495].

Additional studies relating the level of physical activity to the development of coronary heart disease in indoor versus outdoor workers, skilled versus unskilled workers, and athletes versus non-athletes, have demonstrated similar results (Fox and Skinner, 1964). The influence and enthusiasm of the late Dr. Paul Dudley White of Boston were of particular importance in fostering widespread interest on the part of both the public and the medical profession in health, exercise, and fitness programs (White, 1972).

Writers, poets, and those in public life frequently express the interests and concerns of the society in which they live, as the following well-known quotations indicate:

That shows how exercise and self-control enable a man to preserve a great deal of his former strength even after he has become old [Cicero, 44 B.C., p. 226].

Better to hunt in fields for health unbought
Than fee the doctor for a nauseous draught.
The wise for cure on exercise depend;
God never made his work for man to mend.
                    [Dryden, 1700, p. 785]

Those who think they have not time for bodily exercise will sooner or later have to find time for illness [Stanley, 1873].

Unlearn'd, he knew no schoolman's subtle art,
No language but the language of the heart.
By Nature honest, by Experience wise,
Healthy by Temp'rance, and by Exercise.
                    [Pope, n.d., p. 181]

Present-day medical practice builds on the wisdom of the ages in providing a rational approach to exercise for the purpose of maintaining good health and, when necessary, for treating the sick.

20

Rats, Cattle, Spoiled Hay, and Anticoagulants

OVER the past four to five decades, anticoagulants have been used extensively for treating clotting problems in patients with embolic diseases, transient ischemic attacks, venous thromboembolic diseases, valvular heart diseases, and myocardial infarction. The discovery and development of these medications in the years preceding their clinical application have an unusual and interesting history, touched upon briefly in another chapter in describing the medicinal leech and the isolation from this parasitic worm of the first naturally occurring anticoagulant to be reported—hirudin. However, there was little clinical interest at the time of its discovery in developing this latter substance further.

Although coagulant and anticoagulant factors from body tissues were described during the late nineteenth and early twentieth centuries, Jay McLean, a medical student at the John Hopkins University, is usually credited with having made the initial discovery that prepared the way for the eventual development of a clinically useful anticoagulant preparation (1916). Many years later, McLean, reminiscing, recalled that on transferring from the University of California to Johns Hopkins Medical School in Baltimore, he obtained permission to engage in a research project for a year before resuming his regular medical studies (1959). Dr. William Howell, Professor of Physiology, assigned him the task of isolating and purifying the thromboplastic (blood-clotting) factor present in a crude cephalin-containing brain extract. Material from the heart and liver was similarly examined. On working with these substances, McLean noted an interesting phenomenon—that as the stored samples of these materials were periodically re-examined, their blood-clotting activities decreased. Furthermore, as this was occurring, the same samples began to show an opposite and unexpected effect—an ability to prevent coagulation of blood—thus suggesting the presence of an additional substance or factor that had not previously been recognized. This crucial finding was briefly described by McLean in a publication (1916) ironically entitled "The thromboplastic action of cephalin." Two years later, Howell and Holt designated this new anticoagulant factor "as *heparin* to indicate its origin from liver" (1918, p. 328), adding the following comments:

> When freed from mixture with cephalin, a result most difficult to accomplish, this substance [heparin] had a very marked inhibiting effect upon coagulation of blood. . . . The main obstacle [in preparing heparin] lies in the fact that the solubilities of heparin and cephalin are so similar that there is great difficulty in separating them. But until the cephalin or cephalin-like material is removed the properties of the heparin, so far as coagulation is concerned, are masked or antagonized [1918, p. 329].

The difficulties in preparing this anticoagulant so that it could be used clinically came to the attention of Charles Best, co-discoverer of insulin and at that time Assistant Director of the Connaught Laboratories in Toronto. During the 1930s, two of his colleagues, David Scott and Arthur Charles, developed a method for preparing heparin from beef liver (Charles and Scott, 1933) and described procedures for obtaining purer and more active preparations of this material (Scott and Charles, 1933). Clinical application of heparin rapidly followed as it became commercially available. The heart-lung machine used in heart surgery, and the artificial kidney, owe much of their success to the development of this drug and its ability to prevent blood from clotting. Several studies demonstrated the effectiveness of heparin in preventing and treating thrombotic diseases (Crafoord, 1937; Murray, Jaques, Perrett, and Best, 1937; Solandt and Best, 1938), and the drug soon became standard therapy in the management of such problems. Since heparin in of benefit only when given parenterally, much of the discussion about the drug has centered around techniques of administration and dosage—high dose or low dose, continuous or intermittent therapy, and how heparin could best be used in conjunction with other forms of antithrombotic therapy.

It was evident that physicians would welcome an anticoagulant that their patients could take by mouth. Indeed, while studies on heparin were in progress, the first steps along the circuitous route leading to an oral anticoagulant were being made, although those involved were probably unaware of the implications of their work at the time.

In the early 1920s, a mysterious disease of cattle was reported in Canada by veterinarians. In a seminal publication, Frank Schofield, a pathologist at Ontario Veterinary College, described the symptoms and morbid anatomy of these afflicted animals and evaluated the etiologic factors that may have been involved. His conclusions about this new disease, particularly as they relate to later investigations, are well worth citing:

> 1. That the disease investigated is a new disease, and, while simulating hemorrhagic septicemia and blackleg, is entirely distinct from these diseases.
> 2. That the disease is produced by a toxic substance which is present in mouldy sweet clover. There is much evidence that certain moulds are responsible for the formation of this poisonous principle.
> 3. That the toxic substance produces the disease by destroying or damaging the cells of important tissues and vital organs. This may result in hemorrhage, delayed coagulation of the blood, and destruction of the red blood cells.
> 4. That there is no evidence to show that the feeding of good, sweet-clover hay or ensilage can produce the disease in question [1924, pp. 571–572].

Several years later, Lee Roderick, a veterinarian in North Dakota, confirmed that the feeding of damaged or spoiled sweet clover hay caused animals to die of hemorrhage, adding that "the delayed coagulability of the blood in sweet clover disease involves a reduction in the prothrombin and that the diminution parallels the delay in the coagulation time" (1931, p. 424).

Further work on this disease now shifted from Canada and North Dakota to the University of Wisconsin in Madison, where in the mid-1930s, Karl Paul Link and his research team were engaged in isolating and crystallizing the anticoagulant present in spoiled hay, and in developing a bioassay that would measure the anticoagulant activity of the materials they were testing. Various methods for determining prothrombin activity had been devised (Quick, Stanley-Brown, and Bancroft, 1935; Quick, 1937), with the Quick one-stage method adapted by Link and his associates for their experiments. Needless to say, the work was difficult and tedious, but by the early 1940s, Campbell and

Link (1941) had isolated the hemorrhagic agent from spoiled hay in the pure state, and Stahmann, Huebner, and Link (1941) had synthesized this substance and identified it as 3,3'-methylenebis(4-hydroxycoumarin), subsequently called dicumarol; they also demonstrated that the synthetic and the naturally occurring products were chemically identical and biologically equal.

Soon after its isolation, preliminary reports describing the use of dicumarol in thrombotic diseases appeared in the medical literature, stimulating studies that in some instances would continue for many years (Bingham, Meyer, and Pohle, 1941; Allen, Barker, and Waugh, 1942; Dale and Jaques, 1942; Wright and Prandoni, 1942).

The spin-off from the saga of sick cattle, damaged or spoiled sweet clover, and anticoagulants was not yet complete. In the process of identifying dicumarol, many other coumarins had been synthesized and categorized by number. Link became interested in rodent control and felt that one of these coumarin derivatives might be suitable for this purpose. It had been noted that unlike other poisons which a rat would eventually recognize and stop eating, the animal appeared unable to detect coumarin compounds in its food and thus would continue to eat coumarin-laced bait until death from internal bleeding. Coumarin derivative No. 42 was tested, proved to be a satisfactory poison, and early in 1948 was promoted for rodent control under the auspices of the Wisconsin Alumni Research Foundation. Link later explained, "The name Warfarin [for this rodenticide] was coined by me by combining the first letters of the Wisconsin Alumni Research Foundation with the "arin" from coumarin—and it is now a household word throughout the world" (1959, p. 104).

Not long after warfarin was introduced as a rat poison, Holmes and Love (1952) described a patient who took the material in an attempted suicide attempt. This unusual incident, according to Link, "acted as a catalyst" (1959, p. 105) that eventually led to warfarin—the rat poison—replacing dicumarol as the medically prescribed anticoagulant of choice in the United States. The new agent was marketed under the trade name *Coumadin*.

In recent years, there has been increasing use of antiplatelet drugs (aspirin, dipyridamole, sulfinpyrazone) and of thrombolytic agents (streptokinase, tissue plasminogen activator) in preventing and treating thrombotic diseases. It remains to be seen, however, whether accounts of these or any future drugs in this field will ever be able to match this unusual story of the anticoagulants in which an acceptable medical therapy was the unexpected outcome of a saga that had a fatal disease of cattle and a poison for rats as landmarks along the way.

21

Rauwolfia Serpentina, Snakebites, and Hypertension

R AUWOLFIA SERPENTINA—sometimes called the snakeroot plant
because of its long tapering snakelike roots—is native to Ceylon,
the East Indies, and India. As per Linnaeus's original spelling in the
botanical nomenclature, the genus of the plant is given as *Rauvolfia,*
whereas *Rauwolfia*—with a *w*—is the commonly accepted spelling for
those in pharmaceutical practice and in other nonbotanical sciences.
The confusing historical details "of the variant orthographies" of this
plant have been explained by Woodson, Youngken, Schlittler, and
Schneider (1957, pp. 5–6).

Over the centuries, the plant has been used as a popular folk
medicine in India, where it was known by such diverse names as
"*sarpagandha* in Sanskrit, referring to its use as an antidote for snake
bite; *chandra* in Hindi, meaning 'moon' and alluding to its calming
effect upon lunacy. . . . [and] *pagal-ke-dawa,* the insanity herb"
(Kreig, 1964, p. 319). The comprehensive and monumental works of
Charaka in medicine and Sushruta (Susruta) in surgery two thousand
or more years ago "refer to the use of rauwolfia . . . in a large number
of conditions like snake bite, scorpion and insect bite, epilepsy, fevers,
malaria and or course, insanity too" (Dikshit, 1980, p. IX). In addition,
according to sources cited by Monachino, the plant was also used as
a remedy for dysentery and other intestinal disorders, and as an agent
to promote childbirth (1954, p. 350).

Rauwolfia as a genus of plants was named in 1703 by the French
botanist Charles Plumier in honor of Leonhard (Leonard) Rauwolf,
a sixteenth-century physician, botanist, and explorer from Augsberg,

155

Germany. Over fifty years later, in 1755, a book by Georg Eberhardt
Rumpf entitled *Herbarium Amboinense* contained what is said to be
the first known illustration of *Rauwolfia serpentina*. A few passages
from this work describing the legendary background of the plant and
some of its benefits, particularly in snakebites, have been excerpted
by Kreig:

> Men seem to have learned the powers of this plant [the snakeroot] from
> the so-called mongoose or weasel. This little animal, before attacking a snake,
> fortifies itself by eating the leaves [of the plant]; or, if injured in combat with
> a snake, seeks out this herb, eats the leaves, rolls itself around three or four
> times, then rests a little as if drugged, but soon afterwards regains its strength
> and rushes forward to re-attack. It is used for the following diseases: The natives
> of Bengal and Malabar say that the root ground in water produces a decoction
> that is an outstanding antidote against any poison that causes the body to swell
> and grow blue. . . . Freshly pounded roots and leaves may be placed under
> the toe-nails. . . . When the stalks are broken, a milky juice exudes. This is
> instilled in the eyes to remove the white spots or opacities. In Batavia, the plant
> is used thus: The root is cut into small pieces and swallowed; this is of value
> in cases of anxiety and of pain in the stomach. When finely ground up and
> drunk in water, the root is also of value in fever and vomiting, likewise for
> headache if the head is washed with a decoction. It is said to cure the bite of
> most poisonous snakes, even the Cobra *capella* [1964, pp. 319–320].

Dr. Gananath Sen and Dr. Kartick Chandra Bose from Calcutta,
India, in one of the earliest published reports on the use of *Rauwolfia*
(*Rawolfia*) *serpentina* for the treatment of high blood pressure, intro-
duced their discussion as follows:

> With those who know the drug and use it in insanity, it is usually a
> precious and closely guarded secret. . . .
> The first author was fortunate in discovering the effect of the drug in Blood
> Pressure also, and he was able to regulate the blood pressure of his patients
> with the aid of this valuable and safe weapon in his armamentarium almost
> to a precision not found possible with any other drug, Eastern and Western
> [1931, p. 194].

Although confirming the benefits of the drug in psychiatric disorders, Sen and Bose cautioned that treatment was "effective only in
a certain type of insanity which is common. Insanity with violent
maniacal symptoms yield [*sic*] readily to it [rauwolfia]. . . . In the
demented and morose type of insanity, R. Serpentina is not effective,
it is rather contra-indicated" (1931, p. 201). In addition, the drug had
"a very marked depressing action on the sexual centres" (p. 200).

Having noted that extracts of the drug lowered blood pressure by means of vasodilatation and probably by a depressant action on heart muscle, the authors discussed in greater detail their results in treating hypertensive patients:

> R. Serpentina is a very effective remedy when it is used cautiously in regulated doses. It is best suited for the plethoric and nervous type without much atheroma of the blood-vessels. . . . in doses of 5 to 20 grs. given daily, the effect was very striking, even when the diet was not cut down too much. Such symptoms as headache, sense of heat and insomnia disappeared quickly and the blood-pressure was reduced from, say, 200 to 160 within a week or two. In their trials on several hundred patients extending over 3 years the authors have found that a slow reduction of blood-pressure with the sole aid of this drug in small doses was the best way of treating cases of high blood-pressure [1931, p. 201].

This publication by Sen and Bose concluded with the hope and request "that medical men all over the world would work out the effect of this remedy both pharmacologically and clinically as it promises to be a valuable addition to the aramamentarium [*sic*] of the physician" (p. 201). However, their appeal appeared to stimulate little response outside of India until almost twenty years later, when a report about the drug was published in the *British Heart Journal* by Dr. Rustom Jal Vakil, an Indian physician. Stating that he had "found R. *Serpentina* to be the most consistently successful member of the whole group of hypotensive remedies" (1949, p. 350), Vakil described his observations on fifty patients during antihypertensive treatment with tablets made from the dried roots of this plant:

> After four weeks of R. *Serpentina* therapy, 85 percent of cases displayed a drop of systolic blood pressure varying from 2 to 54 mm. with an average of 21 mm. . . .
> In 81 per cent of cases, the diastolic pressure showed a drop of 4 to 34 mm. with an average of 11 mm. . . .
> . . . Amongst the few unpleasant symptoms encountered during its [the medication's] administration, were excessive drowsiness (in 12 per cent), lassitude (in 8 per cent), diarrhoea (in 6 per cent), anorexia (in 4 per cent) and nausea with vomiting (in 4 per cent) [1949, p. 355].

Taking note of this and prior publications in the Indian medical literature, Robert Wilkins in Boston designed a series of studies during the early 1950s to further evaluate the response of patients to these rauwolfia preparations. Confirming much of the previous work from India, Wilkins made the following additional observations:

It [rauwolfia] causes sedation, bradycardia, hypotension, nasal stuffiness, weight gain, and, in excessive doses, diarrhoea, nightmares and agitated depression. It does not cause postural hypotension, and is not narcotic even in large doses [1954, p. 89].

While affirming that "these preparations may find their chief usefulness in many psychoneuroses and tension states, in addition to hypertension" (1954, p. 88), Wilkins also commented, somewhat prophetically, that "Rauwolfia is certainly a valuable addition to our armamentarium against hypertension, not so much because it is a powerful or striking hypotensive agent (which it is not) as because . . . it acts very well in combination with other more powerful drugs" (1953, p. 1304).

In spite of its demonstrated effectiveness as an antihypertensive drug and as a tranquilizing agent, the publications from India and from Wilkins in the United States contained many disturbing hints and suggestions that rauwolfia preparations would eventually have a limited role in medical practice. Although initially they were used with enthusiasm—and what medication is not?—an increasing number of significant dose-related side effects began to be reported, including depression with suicidal potential, gastrointestinal symptoms related to increased gastric acid secretion and ulcer formation, and numerous less threatening but nevertheless troubling problems such as lassitude, nasal stuffiness, weight gain, and impotence, a group of symptoms that would strongly influence patient compliance in taking the medication. In the face of these adverse drug effects, and with the advent of newer and more effective antihypertensive and tranquilizing drugs, the use of rauwolfia preparations has been curtailed in the United States, leading to the comment by Weiner in a leading pharmacology textbook: "Because of the severity of the dose-related side effects of reserpine [a purified alkaloid isolated from *Rauwolfia serpentina*], the drug is administered in low doses and is used only in conjunction with other types of antihypertensive agents" (1985, p. 210).

By recognizing and using clues about medical therapies from the past, as, for example, the references to the effects of rauwolfia in ancient Hindu medical lore, researchers have often been able to expand upon present-day knowledge and medical practices. Even if an ancient remedy proves to be of only transient use, it may often serve as a useful stepping stone to further discoveries. Rauwolfia has served such a valuable purpose.

22

Nitroglycerine: An Old Favorite
with New Tricks

A NY discussion of nitroglycerine and related medications would be incomplete without reference to the disorder for which these remedies were intended—angina pectoris. The classic and oft-quoted description of the symptoms experienced by those so afflicted was written by William Heberden (1710–1801) approximately two centuries ago and published posthumously in his *Commentaries on the History and Cure of Diseases*. This account is as valid today as it was at that time:

> But there is a disorder of the breast marked with strong and peculiar symptoms, considerable for the kind of danger belonging to it, and not extremely rare, which deserves to be mentioned more at length. The seat of it, and sense of strangling, and anxiety with which it is attended, may make it not improperly be called angina pectoris.
>
> They who are afflicted with it, are seized while they are walking, (more especially if it be up hill, and soon after eating) with a painful and most disagreeable sensation in the breast, which seems as if it would extinguish life, if it were to increase or to continue; but the moment they stand still, all this uneasiness vanishes [1802, pp. 363–364].

Typical episodes of angina pectoris may occur during physical exertion, emotional stress, or exposure to cold weather, activities which add to the work of the heart and thus increase its requirements for oxygen beyond the ability of the coronary blood flow to keep pace. Nitroglycerine and related compounds relax smooth muscle in the walls of systemic arteries and veins and by so doing cause these vessels to dilate. This decreases both the amount of blood returning to the heart and the resistance against which the heart has to operate. As a

161

consequence of these hemodynamic alterations, the work of the heart and its oxygen requirements are reduced. At the same time, regional myocardial (heart muscle) blood flow is improved by the action of these medications upon coronary arteries. The effect of this medical therapy, therefore, is to reverse many of the pathophysiologic changes that occur in angina pectoris and to modify the patient's symptoms. The series of empirical observations and clinical studies that led over the years to the current use of these medications for cardiac disorders is a fascinating part of medical history that, like the story of many forms of medical treatment, has strange twists and turns.

Thomas Lauder Brunton (1844–1916) was born in Scotland and attended the University of Edinburgh for his medical studies. He settled in London, where he eventually became full physician at St. Bartholomew's Hospital, making many notable contributions to the medical literature. However, it was during his early years as resident physician at the Royal Infirmary in Edinburgh prior to moving to London that Brunton published his well-known article on the use of amyl nitrite in patients with angina pectoris. The introduction to this work is a masterfully worded statement reflecting the author's raison d'être for initiating the study:

> Few things are more distressing to a physician than to stand beside a suffering patient who is anxiously looking to him for that relief from pain which he feels himself utterly unable to afford. His sympathy for the sufferer, and the regret he feels for the impotence of his art, engrave the picture indelibly on his mind, and serve as a constant and urgent stimulus in his search after the causes of the pain, and the means by which it may be alleviated.
>
> Perhaps there is no class of cases in which such occurrences as this take place so frequently as in some kinds of cardiac disease, in which angina pectoris forms at once the most prominent and the most painful and distressing symptom [1867, p. 97].

Brunton continued his report with a brief review of the pertinent although limited information then available on amyl nitrite, explaining how prior studies had led him to believe that this medication might be of benefit in patients with angina pectoris:

> Nitrite of amyl was discovered by Balard; and further investigated by Guthrie, who noticed its property of causing flushing of the face, throbbing of the carotids, and acceleration of the heart's action, and proposed it as a resuscitative in drowning, suffocation, and protracted fainting.
>
> Little attention, however, was paid to it for some years, till it was again taken up by Dr. B. W. Richardson, who found that it caused paralysis of the

nerves from the periphery inwards, diminished the contractility of muscles, and caused dilatation of the capillaries, as seen in the web of the frog's foot.

Dr. Arthur Gamgee, in an unpublished series of experiments both with the sphygmograph and haemadynamometer, has found that it [amyl nitrite] greatly lessens the arterial tension both in animals and man; and it was these experiments—some of which I was fortunate enough to witness—which led me to try it in angina pectoris [1867, p. 97].

Several patients with this disorder were described by Brunton in whom the usual remedies of the time such as digitalis, aconite, and lobelia inflata gave no relief. The author made the interesting observation that

[s]mall bleedings of three or four ounces, whether by cupping or venesection, were, however, always beneficial. . . . As I believed the relief produced by the bleeding to be due to the diminution it occasioned in the arterial tension, it occurred to me that a substance which possesses the power of lessening it in such an eminent degree as nitrite of amyl would probably produce the same effect, and might be repeated as often as necessary without detriment to the patient's health [1867, p. 98].

Brunton also noted that during an attack of angina "the pulse becomes smaller, and the arterial tension greater as the pain increases in severity" (1867, p. 98). Thus, from these and other related clinical observations and from his knowledge of amyl nitrite, Brunton reasoned that the drug might be useful in reversing the acute physiological changes in angina pectoris and in alleviating the symptoms of this disorder. Indeed, "On pouring from five to ten drops of the nitrite on a cloth and giving it to the patient to inhale, the physiological action took place in from thirty to sixty seconds; and simultaneously with the flushing of the face the pain completely disappeared" (p. 98).

An interesting aside to this story is that Brunton reportedly used amyl nitrite to terminate episodes of angina that he himself was experiencing (Krantz, 1975, p. 5).

The development of nitroglycerine as a remedy for angina pectoris lagged only slightly in time behind that of amyl nitrite. Priority for the preparation of a series of nitrated explosives, including nitroglycerine, was claimed by Sobrero in a letter published in 1847 (Munch and Petter, 1965, p. 491). An editorial appearing in a German journal, the *Annalen der Chemie und Pharmacie*, described this work, concluding that "a little of it [nitroglycerine] put on the tongue brings about a persisting migraine [headache]. . . . By heating it, the substance is detonated" (*Annalen der Chemie und Pharmacie*, 1848, p. 398). The latter feature was exploited by the Swedish engineer Alfred B. Nobel, the creator of the Nobel prizes, in producing dynamite. The former characteristic, a headache, is part of the saga of nitroglycerine, the medication, as later noted by many other observers.

Shortly thereafter, the report on Sobrero's new substance apparently came to the attention of Professor Constantin Hering at the Hahnemann Medical School in Philadelphia. In conjunction with Morris Davis, a chemist, a limited quantity of this "desired product" (Munch and Petter, 1965, p. 491) was obtained. Small doses were found to be extremely potent, and in order to develop a more standardized and dependable dosage form of the minute amounts needed, "the new product was dissolved in alcohol and the solution was absorbed by sugar pellets, each pellet containing from 1/300th to 1/5000th drop. These treated sugar pellets were then administered sublingually" (p. 491). A sublingual form of nitroglycerine has persisted in common usage to the present-day.

Since this material had not been analyzed nor given a suitable name, Hering took the initial letters of the components that formed this substance—*G*lycyl *O*xide and *N*itrogen and *O*xygen—and in the manner of an acrostic, and by adding a suitable suffix, called it *glonoin* (Munch and Petter, 1965, p. 494). It was proposed "that this new product should be helpful in the treatment of coronary involvements, angina pectoris, cardiac edema, headache [*sic*], epilepsy and cerebral involvements, among other disease conditions" (Munch and Petter, 1965, p. 494). A few years later, Field described his experience with this new medication, stating that he was introduced to it by a homeopathic practitioner, "an enthusiastic disciple of Hahnemann" (1858, p. 291). After swallowing a small quantity himself, Field wrote that he

experienced a sensation of fulness in both sides of the neck, to this succeeded nausea, and I said "I shall be sick." The next sensation of which I was conscious was, as if some of the same fluid was being poured down my throat, and then succeeded a few moments of uncertainty as to where I was, during which there was a loud rushing noise in my ears, like steam passing out of a tea-kettle, and a feeling of constriction around the lower part of my neck as if my coat were buttoned too tightly; my forehead was wet with perspiration, and I yawned frequently [1858, p. 291).

A smaller dose apparently caused a somewhat less alarming and less violent reaction with Field noting "a sense of constriction of the neck, slight nausea, with fulness, and some pain in the head, as if the brain were expanding" (p. 291). In spite of these reactions, Field administered the medication to several patients, only one of whom may possibly have had symptoms of angina pectoris, commenting enthusiastically, "I have not yet met with one well-defined case of neuralgic or spasmodic disease in which this medicine has failed to afford relief" (p. 292).

It remained, however, for William Murrell (1853–1912), associated for much of his professional life with Westminster Hospital in London, to make the significant observations that eventually resulted in the clinical use of this new medication, now known as nitroglycerine, in patients with angina pectoris. Murrell noted that previous investigators had described a variety of different symptoms and effects after taking this substance, and

> being quite at a loss to reconcile the conflicting statements of the different observers, or arrive at any conclusion respecting the properties of the drug, I determined to try its action on myself. . . . I experienced a violent pulsation in my head, and Mr. Field's observations rose considerably in my estimation. The pulsation rapidly increased, and soon became so severe that each beat of the heart seemed to shake my whole body. . . . I took my own pulse, and found that it was much fuller than natural, and considerably over 100. The pulsation was tremendous, and I could feel the beating to the very tips of my fingers. The pen I was holding was violently jerked with every beat of the heart . . . a splitting headache remained for the whole afternoon [1879a, p. 81].

Murrell administered the medication to several other people, noting that they were affected in much the same way. He then drew the following conclusion:

> From a consideration of the physiological action of the drug, and more especially from the similarity existing between its general action and that of nitrite of amyl [as noted by Brunton previously], I concluded that it would probably prove of service in the treatment of angina pectoris, and I am happy to say that this anticipation has been realized [1879b, p. 113].

By means of a series of sphygmographic tracings comparing the effects of nitroglycerine and amyl nitrite, Murrell further demonstrated that although both substances increase the pulse rate and alter the pulse form in similar fashion,

[t]hey differ, however, in the time they respectively take to produce these effects. The full action of the nitro-glycerine is not observed in the sphygmographic tracings until six or seven minutes after the dose has been taken. In the case of nitrite of amyl the effect is obtained in from fifteen to twenty seconds after an inhalation or a dose has been taken on sugar. The influence of the nitrite of amyl is extremely transitory, a tracing taken a minute and a half after the exhibition of the drug being perfectly normal. In fact, the full effect of the nitrite of amyl on the pulse is not maintained for more than fifteen seconds. The nitro-glycerine produces its effects much more slowly; they last longer, and disappear gradually, the tracing not resuming its normal condition for nearly half an hour [1879b, p. 113].

Two additional reports by Murrell (1879c, 1879d) described the benefits of nitroglycerine in several patients with angina pectoris. The inconvenience of inhaling amyl nitrite combined with its transitory effects eventually resulted in nitroglycerine, with its longer and more predictable course of action and its easier route of administration, becoming the preferred agent for the symptomatic management of patients with this disorder. However, citations referring to the use of amyl nitrite were still found in textbooks of the mid-twentieth century written by the well-known cardiologists Paul Dudley White (1944, p. 833) and Paul Wood (1956, pp. 717–718).

Sublingual nitroglycerine has been a reliable friend to both patients and physicians for alleviating the acute symptoms of angina pectoris, for reducing the frequency of such attacks, and for treating heart failure. In addition, various new formulations of this medication have become available in recent years, permitting an individualized and often more appropriate treatment of specific cardiac syndromes. These new preparations include oral forms, both short-acting and time-released; chewable forms; cutaneous or topical preparations administered as an ointment or contained in a reservoir that permits a gradual absorption of the drug over a period of hours—the transdermal patch; a rapidly acting oral spray; a transbuccal preparation that is inserted under the upper lip to allow a slow and uniform release of the medication; and intravenous preparations. Thus, by taking full advantage of the pharmacologic actions of nitroglycerine, and with the aid of additional ways of administering the drug to the patient, the use of an old favorite has been extended to the treatment of a wider spectrum of cardiac problems.

23

Quinidine Therapy: The Countess, Fevers, and Fluttering Hearts

OVER 350 years ago, during the early seventeenth century, an Augustinian monk named Calancha reported in a religious text that the bark of a native tree growing in his region of South America was a miraculous cure for certain types of febrile illnesses (Webster, 1985, p. 1041). During this same period, according to a romanticized account that has become a popular legend in medicine, the Countess of Chinchon, then living in Peru, where her husband was Viceroy, became severely ill, probably with malaria. Cured with the aid of a medication obtained from the bark of a tree, the Countess was subsequently said to have brought this remedy back to Spain with her (Haggis, 1941; Clendening, 1943). In recent years, Haggis (1941), in the role of historical sleuth, has found inconsistencies that cast doubt upon certain details of this tale. Be that as it may, regardless of whether the story is apocryphal, or whether it was the Count or the Countess of Chinchon, merchants, or Jesuit priests who actually introduced the bark into Europe during the seventeenth century, this new cure—called Jesuit's bark or Peruvian bark—became much sought after. Its use was advocated by such individuals as the controversial Robert Talbor in England (Siegel and Poynter, 1962) and the famous Thomas Sydenham (Sydenham, 1676), who recognized that certain fevers, specifically those related to malaria, responded to this medication. Sydenham wrote:

> In regard to the care of quartans [a fever recurring every fourth day], those who are in the least degree conversant with medicine know how unsatisfactory are all those methods which have been designed for the cure of this *opprobrium*

medicorum, Peruvian bark only excepted. Even this checks rather than conquers
them [1676, p. 84].

Recognizing the intermittency of the disease, Sydenham also
indicated that

the powder must be repeated at short intervals, so that the first dose may not
have lost its effect before the exhibition of a second. . . .
    Upon this ground I prefer the following form to any other: Mix one ounce
of Peruvian bark with two of the syrup of red roses, of which the patient must
take a bolus, of the size of a nutmeg, night and morning [1676, p. 85].

Linné, or Linnaeus, the well-known Swedish botanist of the eighteenth century, probably fostered the story of the Countess of Chinchon
by naming this species of plant *cinchona* in her honor (Haggis, 1941),
although according to others this term may have been derived from
a word of Incan origin meaning "bark" (Webster, 1985, p. 1041).

For many years, preparations of cinchona extracts were used as
antipyretic agents in the management of fevers, regardless of their
cause, and as stomachics, remedies to stimulate the stomach and
digestive functions. Although recognizing that the most important use
of this drug was for the treatment of malaria, a pharmacology textbook
of the late nineteenth century by Bartholow indicated that "there can
be no doubt of the good effects in practice of quinia [an alkaloid
obtained from cinchona] in *septicaemia, pyaemia, erysipelas*, and *puer-
peral fever.*" (1882, p. 168). The same author noted that "preparations
of cinchona are much used as stomachic tonics. In *atonic dyspepsia*
they are employed, like the simple bitters, to promote the flow of
gastric juice" (p. 166), adding that "the use of quinia as a restorative
tonic in cases of *debility* is almost universal" (p. 167). The widespread
application of cinchona derivatives in a variety of ailments even extended to a contribution by the great nineteenth-century physicist
Hermann von Helmholtz, who recommended applying quinine sulphate to the nasal mucous membrane in hay fever (Garrison, 1929,
p. 533). As recently as 1947, the twenty-fourth edition of *The Dispensatory of the United States of America*, aside from discussing the
use of quinine in malaria, still contained references to the medication
as an analgesic for headache and myalgia, a stomachic appetizer, and
an antipyretic, and even suggested that the drug could be used to
prevent symptoms of colds and of whooping cough (Osol and Farrar,
1947, pp. 957–961).

One of the earliest references to the use of quinine for treating a cardiac symptom, specifically palpitations, was recorded in 1749 by Jean-Baptiste de Sénac (1693–1770), chief physician to Louis XV of France, in his well-known textbook devoted to the anatomy, physiology, and diseases of the heart. According to Sénac, as cited by Willius and Keys, "The stomachic remedies have appeared to various physicians as a resource against palpitations for it is often in the stomach that their cause resides" (1942, p. 295). It was for this purpose that Sénac apparently recommended the use of quinine: "Of all the stomachic remedies the one whose effects have appeared to me the most constant and the most prompt in many cases, is Quinine mixed with a little rhubarb. Long and rebellious palpitations have ceded to this febrifuge, seconded with a light purgative" (p. 296).

In 1820, Pelletier and Caventou isolated quinine from cinchona (Webster, 1985, p. 1042), allowing physicians to utilize a pure cinchona alkaloid preparation rather than relying on powders, extracts, and infusions of the bark. Another cinchona alkaloid was identified shortly after the middle of the nineteenth century, to which Louis Pasteur later gave the name quinidine (Kay, 1966).

Over the next few years, sporadic references to the cardiac effects of quinine and quinidine appeared in the medical literature. Bartholow wrote that quinia "affects the rate of movement of the heart. . . . [O]rdinary medicinal doses of quinia (from two to five grains) increase the action of the heart, while experiments with large doses have demonstrated that this agent depresses the circulation" (1882, p. 162). In an article published in the *Lancet* entitled "Quinine as a cardiac stimulant," Hare commented that

> observations seemed to point to an action [of quinine] on the heart independent of the antipyresis. . . .
> The effect on the pulse is not limited to a reduction in frequency; the beats become stronger, more sustained, and more distinct, and the change is especially striking in a case where the pulse has been inclined to "run" [1891, p. 930].

Several years later, Karl F. Wenckebach of Vienna wrote that it was the practice of some physicians to add "quinin to digitalis to prevent or relieve the disagreeable action of this drug on the stomach" (1923, p. 472), an apparent example of the longstanding use of quinine as a stomachic rather than an antiarrhythmic medication. Of greater interest is a story referring to an early experience that Wenckebach had with one of his patients who was taking quinine, a lighthearted story that needs to be quoted at length in order to appreciate both its humor and relevance:

> In 1912, a patient presented himself in my office wishing to get rid of his attacks of auricular fibrillation. . . . He did not feel great discomfort during the attack but, as he said, being a Dutch merchant, used to good order in his affairs, he would like to have good order in his heart business also and asked why there were heart specialists if they could not abolish this very disagreeable phenomenon. On my telling him that I could promise him nothing, he told me that he knew himself how to get rid of his attacks, and as I did not believe him he promised to come back the next morning with a regular pulse, and he did. It happens that quinin in many countries, especially in countries where there is a good deal of malaria, is a sort of drug for everything, just as one takes acetylsalicylic acid [aspirin] today if one does not feel well or is afraid of having taken cold. Occasionally, taking the drug during an attack of fibrillation, the patient found that the attack was stopped within from twenty to twenty-five minutes, and later he found that a gram of quinin regularly abolished his irregularity.
>
> I was greatly struck by this fact, and afterward tried this sort of treatment in many cases of auricular fibrillation. My success was disappointing, in that quinin abolished auricular fibrillation in only a few cases and in those cases only when the onset of this form was quite recent, never when it was of several years' duration. At the same time, I found that even in those cases in which auricular fibrillation was not abolished, the drug had a marked soothing action on the often terrific rate of the ventricle [Wenckebach, 1923, p. 472].

Between 1918 and 1921, Frey in Germany observed that quinidine was more successful than quinine in restoring normal heart rhythm in subjects with auricular fibrillation (White, Marvin, and Burwell, 1921). Previous work by Lewis, Drury, Iliescu, and Wedd had demonstrated "that in auricular fibrillation a circus movement exists in the auricle; that a single wave is propagated and revolves perpetually upon a re-entrant path" (1921, p. 514). Quinidine is successful in bringing "fibrillation of the auricle to an end" (p. 514), these authors noted, because it

> prolongs the refractory period of the auricle and delays the recovery of the tissue, thus rendering the gap between the crest and the wake of the circulating wave shorter and eventually abolishing it altogether; when the last event happens the abnormal action of the auricle ceases and the normal impulses are thus enabled once again to resume control [1921, p. 514].

However, quinidine was also shown to have another action, that of slowing the rate of conduction, thus tending to perpetuate rather than abolish the circus movement in the auricle. Whichever of these two actions of quinidine predominated would, according to Lewis et al., determine whether or not the arrhythmia was converted to a normal heart rhythm. These authors, therefore, advised caution in administering this medication, noting that quinidine "is a remedy of which we still have much too little knowledge; it is one which, unless it is controlled by frequent records of the auricular and ventricular action, is not without serious risk" (1921, p. 515).

Based upon the combined experiences of a group of well-known physicians called the Cardiac Club, whose original members included Thomas Lewis and John Parkinson, an interesting report from England described the effect of quinidine in 265 patients with auricular fibrillation (Hay, 1924). Nearly 60 percent of these patients converted to a normal heart rhythm following treatment, albeit some only temporarily. Seven of these patients sustained an embolism, and another eight patients receiving quinidine died for unexplained reasons. The author stated that it is unwise to administer quinidine if there is a prior history of embolism or if there is an idiosyncrasy—not specifically defined—to the drug. The recent attention being directed toward the provocation or aggravation of arrhythmias by antiarrhythmic drug therapy itself and the potential life-threatening consequences of this serious complication (Velebit, Podrid, Lown, Cohen, and Graboys, 1982) emphasize the significance of these findings by Hay and recall the previously cited caution expressed by Lewis et al. that the remedy, quinidine, "is not without serious risk" (1921, p. 515).

The use of a medication for a different purpose than originally intended, in this case the antimalarial drug quinine that eventually evolved into the arrhythmic drug quinidine, is an often-told tale in medicine. However, as the story of quinine and quinidine also illustrates, expanded uses of a medication may at times result in the remedy causing additional and unexpected adverse effects, a possibility for which physicians must be constantly on the alert. Thus, it is well to remember Douglas Zipes' comments on present-day therapy for rhythm disturbances of the heart, namely, that "pharmacologic control of arrhythmia still remains predicated on an individual, patient-by-patient, pharmacologic experiment, determined by trial and error, and tempered by good clinical judgment" (1985, p. 955).

24

Beta-Adrenergic Blocking Agents: The Beta Blockers

THE history of beta-adrenergic blocking agents—the beta block-ers—is comparatively short, this form of therapy having been introduced into clinical medicine during the 1960s for the management of cardiac arrhythmias, angina, and hypertension. The conceptual origins of this group of medications, however, extend back many years prior to this time, and incorporate some of the most exciting and original discoveries made in physiology and pharmacology.

The idea that receptor sites are present on cells, and that the chemical transmission of nerve impulses from the autonomic nervous system to these cell receptors could be altered, may be traced to the work of John Langley, Professor of Physiology at Cambridge University. Using curare and nicotine to investigate the properties of the nervous and muscular systems, Langley proposed that "the different systems of efferent nerves would chiefly, at any rate, owe their differences to the different characters of the 'receptive' substances of the cells with which they have become connected" (1906, p. 193). During this same period, Henry Dale at the Wellcome Physiological Research Laboratories, by studying the effects of ergot preparations upon the responses of the sympathetic nervous system, demonstrated that

> ergot contains a principle which has a paralytic action on the motor elements of that myotrophic structure or substance which is excited by adrenaline and by impulses in fibres of the true sympathetic system; the inhibitor elements of the same being relatively or absolutely unaffected [1906, p. 204].

This classic work by Dale demonstrated that the expected pressor response in decerebrate cats following the administration of adrenaline could be prevented or blocked by pretreatment with certain ergot compounds. Almost forty years later, Nickerson and Goodman made a similar observation when another sympatho-adrenal blocking agent was used, noting that the characteristic rise in blood pressure usually seen with an injection of epinephrine was instead followed by a fall in pressure when such an injection was made into an animal pretreated with dibenamine. They stated that "The reversal by Dibenamine of the pressor response to epinephrine probably represents a blocking of the vasoconstrictor action and a consequent unmasking of the inhibitory vasodilator action of epinephrine" (1947, p. 169). A later classification would identify dibenamine as an alpha-adrenergic blocking agent.

Upon the basis of observations such as these, Raymond Ahlquist at the University of Georgia School of Medicine published a landmark article, stating that "although there are two kinds of adrenotropic receptors they cannot be classified simply as excitatory or inhibitory since each kind of receptor may have either action depending upon where it is found" (1948, p. 586). Ahlquist further proposed that instead of there being two different mediator substances, as some had suggested, there were actually two different receptors, called by him alpha and beta adrenotropic receptors, and that the

> *alpha* adrenotropic receptor is associated with most of the excitatory functions (vasoconstriction, and stimulation of the uterus, nictitating membrane, uretur and *dilator pupillae*) and one important inhibitory function (intestinal relaxation). The *beta* adrenotropic receptor is associated with most of the inhibitory functions (vasodilation, and inhibition of the uterine and bronchial musculature) and one excitatory function (myocardial stimulation) [1948, p. 599].

Confirmation of Ahlquist's ideas came from a variety of studies on adrenergic blocking agents. Following the demonstration by Powell and Slater that DCI, a dichloro analogue of isoproterenol, "selectively blocked some inhibitory effects of epinephrine and isoproterenol" (1958, p. 487), Moran and Perkins reported that administration of this agent "selectively blocks the cardiac positive inotropic and chronotropic effects of adrenergic stimuli in dogs" (1958, p. 236), noting the following in their summary remarks:

> On the basis of the selective blockade by DCI of the excitatory effects of adrenergic stimuli on the heart and of their inhibitory effects on other organs

(e.g. the vasodepressor effect of isoproterenol) and the lack of blockade of adrenergic vasopressor action, it is concluded that the adrenergic receptors of mammalian hearts are functionally homologous to the adrenergic inhibitory receptors of other tissues. This conclusion agrees with the hypothesis of Ahlquist that the cardiac inotropic and chronotropic sympathetic receptors are of the *beta* type, receptors which subserve inhibitory functions in other organs, in contrast to the *alpha* receptors which subserve sympathetic excitatory responses in all organs except the heart [1958, p. 236].

Three years later, these same authors referred to this drug as a beta-adrenergic blocking agent, stating that

adrenergic blocking agents be classified on the basis of the type of the adrenotropic receptor which is blocked. According to Ahlquist's classification of adrenergic receptors, DCI would be a *beta* adrenergic blocking drug and the classical agents [ergot alkaloids, dibenamine] would be *alpha* adrenergic blocking drugs [Moran and Perkins, 1961, p. 192].

Dichloroisoproterenol (DCI) was the first compound shown to produce selective blockade of beta-adrenergic receptors—it is, thus, a beta blocker—although it had limited clinical usefulness because of potent sympathomimetic activity, i.e., increasing heart rate. James Black at the Pharmaceuticals Division of Imperial Chemical Industries Ltd. in England wondered whether a beta-adrenergic blocking agent could be found without this intrinsic sympathomimetic activity. If so, it was reasoned, by blocking the action of adrenaline upon heart rate and force of contraction, it might be possible to reduce the demands of the heart for oxygen, thus providing a different approach to treating such disorders as angina pectoris and arrhythmias. By the early 1960s, Black and Stephenson were able to describe a new compound with these properties, stating that nethalide

is an effective antagonist of adrenergic beta receptors.
    This compound blocks the cardiac rate of tension changes produced by catecholamines, but differs from dichloroisoprenaline (D.C.I.) in being free from intrinsic sympathomimetic activity.
    In conscious animals, bradycardia is the most obvious sign of activity of the compound; it is suggested that this is due to myocardial adrenergic blockade [1962, p. 314].

Dornhorst and Robinson at St. George's Hospital in London administered nethalide to human subjects, confirming that the compound "is an effective antagonist of the beta action of catecholamines. . . . The ability of the drug to increase exercise tolerance in our patients with ischaemic heart-disease is encouraging" (1962, p. 316). Of additional interest were the precautionary words at the conclusion of their report regarding the use of this agent in patients with heart failure:

> Reduction of adrenergic cardiac stimulation clearly produces no disability in normal subjects. There is, however, reason to think that in circulatory failure the maintenance of cardiac output may critically depend on neurogenic drive, and in such circumstances great caution will be needed in the use of this and similar drugs [1962, p. 316].

In spite of this problem, the benefits of a new approach to treating cardiac disorders, as voiced initially by Black, were realized. Side effects with nethalide, also called pronethalol, later restricted its use in humans, with toxicity studies demonstrating the appearance of malignant tumors in mice. Within two years after the initial reports on this drug had appeared, however, another compound was identified without these drawbacks. Black, Crowther, Shanks, Smith, and Dornhorst (1964) introduced propranolol to the medical profession, an agent with wider therapeutic potential, less side effects, and without the carcinogenic potential of its forebear.

Rapid accumulation of clinical experience and knowledge about this significantly different approach to the medical treatment of cardiac disorders prompted the presentation of a symposium at Buxton, England, in 1965, attended by internationally prominent physicians, physiologists, and pharmacologists. The papers presented at the meeting were published, serving as an authoritative review and reference for the medical profession. In an introductory editorial to the publication containing these reports, Braunwald prophetically set the future course for this group of drugs:

> [I]t should be evident that exploitation of the differences between beta adrenergic receptors in various tissues might make it possible to block selectively only certain beta adrenergic functions. For example, if an agent were found which would block the beta adrenergic receptors in the sinoatrial node and specialized conduction tissue of the heart without affecting the beta receptors in the ventricular myocardium, then the antiarrhythmic properties of such a drug which are exerted on these tissues might not be limited by its simultaneous removal of sympathetic support to the myocardium. While the papers of this Symposium clearly prove the clinical usefulness of propranolol, it is not unreasonable to hope that this compound will prove to be the prototype of more selective beta adrenergic blocking agents which will play even more decisive roles in the management of a variety of cardiovascular disorders [1966, p. 307].

Within one year of these comments, the beta adrenergic group of receptors had been categorized into two distinct receptor types, beta$_1$ and beta$_2$ (Lands, Arnold, McAuliff, Luduena, and Brown, 1967). In rapid sequence, the discovery of selective beta-blocking agents followed—agents that blocked the beta$_1$ receptors in the heart but not the beta$_2$ receptors elsewhere—thus avoiding undesired effects of treatment and providing the opportunity of tailoring therapy to specific problems. As Julius Comroe, Jr., wrote,

> In essence, pharmaceutical research chemists are now chemically subdividing the sites of action of norepinephrine into smaller and smaller chunks—as far as cell function is concerned—so that the physician now has drugs that can suppress a single function of your bodywide sympathetic nervous system and provide you with a highly specific beneficial effect with less and less chance of undesired drug actions [1983, p. 269].

For their pioneering work in this field, James Black and Raymond Ahlquist received the prestigious Albert Lasker Award in Clinical Research for 1976. James Black was also a recipient of the Nobel Prize for Physiology or Medicine in 1988. The complexities of pharmaceutical research of this type were perhaps put into perspective by Shanks, himself one of the early investigators of beta adrenergic blocking agents, when he wrote that the "successful discovery and commercial development of a new drug depends on the interaction of many factors including original ideas, foresight, intuition, careful scientific observation, integrated chemical and pharmacological effect and luck" (1984, p. 409).

25

Heart Surgery: The Early Years

"A surgeon who tries to suture a heart wound deserves to lose the esteem of his colleagues." According to Johnson (1970, p. 3), this comment was attributed to Theodor Billroth, one of Europe's most famous and respected surgeons during the last half of the nineteenth century, and no doubt reflected the concern of the profession at that time with operations upon the heart. Fortunately, there were those who ignored this warning. Several years after Billroth's comment, Ludwig Rehn, Professor of Surgery at the University of Frankfurt, described the successful repair of a laceration of the right ventricle in a twenty-two year old patient who had received a knife wound of the chest. Rehn's report, entitled "Ueber penetrirende Herzwunden und Herznaht" ("Penetrating cardiac wounds and cardiac suture"), boldly concluded: "The feasibility of a cardiac suture should from now on no longer be held in doubt" (1897, p. 44).

Before heart surgery could be developed further, additional progress had to be made in managing the cardiopulmonary consequences of operating within the chest, particularly the problem of an open pneumothorax. In the early years of the twentieth century, the German surgeon Ferdinand Sauerbruch, aware of the importance of maintaining a negative pressure in the pleural space, devised, according to Graham, "a chamber which actually amounted to a small operating room. The body of the patient and those of the surgeon and his assistants were inside the chamber which had a pressure less than that of the atmosphere and the heads were outside" (1957, p. 241). Although the apparatus was sound in principle for preventing pneumothorax, its cumbersomeness limited its widespread use.

In an ingenious yet simple experiment, Meltzer and Auer of the Rockefeller Institute for Medical Research "discovered the fact that under certain conditions respiration can be carried on by continuous inflation of the lungs, and without any normal or artificial rhythmical respiratory movements whatever" (1909, p. 622). As an outgrowth of this study, the development of insufflation intratracheal anesthesia permitted the pleura to be opened at the time of an operation without fear of a pneumothorax, thus removing a major obstacle to the progress of heart surgery.

Two years before the beginning of the twentieth century, Dr. D. W. Samways wrote: "I anticipate that with the progress of cardiac surgery some of the severest cases of mitral stenosis will be relieved by slightly notching the mitral orifice and trusting to the auricle to continue its defence" (1898, p. 927). Four years later, Sir Lauder Brunton outlined a farsighted and at the time controversial plan for operating upon the mitral valve:

> Mitral stenosis is not only one of the most distressing forms of cardiac disease, but in its severe forms it resists all treatment by medicine. On looking at the contracted mitral orifice in a severe case of this disease one is impressed by the hopelessness of ever finding a remedy which will enable the auricle to drive the blood in a sufficient stream through the small mitral orifice, and the wish unconsciously arises that one could divide the constriction as easily during life as one can after death. The risk which such an operation would entail naturally makes one shrink from it, but in some cases it might be well worth while for the patients to balance the risk of a shortened life against the certainty of a prolonged period of existence which could hardly be called life, as the only conditions under which it could be continued might to them be worse than death [1902, p. 352].

This vivid description, voicing the frustration of one who was trying to treat these patients with medical therapy alone, provided Brunton a framework on which to base a discussion of surgical approaches and methods that could be used to enlarge the valve opening. At the conclusion of this remarkable albeit brief paper, Brunton stated: "The good results that have been obtained by surgical treatment of wounds in the heart emboldens one to hope that before very long similar good results may be obtained in cases of mitral stenosis" (p. 352). How accurately these prophesies by Samways and Brunton were borne out in later years!

During the 1920s, Cutler and Levine at Harvard Medical School and the Peter Bent Brigham Hospital experimented with various procedures for operating upon the stenotic mitral valve, finally deciding "that it seemed wiser to use the simpler and more speedy route through the ventricular wall with the valvulotome [a surgical knife] in the first human case" (1923, p. 1024). The opportunity to apply this surgical approach arose on May 20, 1923, when a young girl with severe mitral stenosis was taken to the operating room, an incision made from the top of the sternum to an area just above the umbilicus, and the heart exposed. Like the reports of those who first flew an airplane or who first reached the summit of Mr. Everest, the verbatim description by those participating in the operation allows the reader to best appreciate the excitement and magic of those next crucial moments:

> This moment was seized as our most propitious one, and rolling the heart out and to the right by the left hand, the valvulotome, an instrument somewhat similar to a tenotome or a slightly curved tonsil knife, and the one with which we were most familiar in our experimental work, was taken in the right hand and plunged into the left ventricle at a point about one inch from the apex and away from the branches of the descended [*sic*] coronary artery, where two mattress sutures had already been placed. The knife was pushed upwards about 2½ inches, until it encountered what seemed to us must be the mitral orifice. It was then turned mesially, and a cut made in what we thought was the aortic leaflet, the resistance encountered being very considerable. The knife was quickly turned and a cut made in the opposite side of the opening. The knife was then withdrawn and the mattress sutures already in place were tied over the point at which the knife had been inserted. There was absolutely no bleeding. Hot saline was dripped onto the heart, whose action continued good [Cutler and Levine, 1923, p. 1025].

The authors added that "recovery was rapid, as it is in most children once the period of convalescence becomes well established. Her appetite, spirits, strength, and general condition responded marvelously. Seven days after operation the sutures and all dressings were removed" (1923, p. 1026).

Henry Souttar at the London Hospital is credited with having established the principles upon which closed mitral valve surgery was later based. On May 6, 1925, using intratracheal anesthesia, Souttar operated upon a nineteen-year-old girl with combined mitral stenosis and regurgitation. Unlike the operation by Cutler and Levine in which the valve was opened blindly with a knife, Souttar performed this procedure with his finger, introducing it into the auricle and across the mitral opening into the ventricle, and actually feeling the valve. He concluded his report as follows:

It appears to me that the method of digital exploration through the auricular appendage cannot be surpassed for simplicity and directness. Not only is the mitral orifice directly to hand, but the aortic valve itself is almost certainly within reach, through the mitral orifice. Owing to the simplicity of the structures, and, oddly enough, to their constant and regular movement, the information given by the finger is exceedingly clear, and personally I felt an appreciation of the mechanical reality of stenosis and regurgitation which I never before possessed. To hear a murmur is a very different matter from feeling the blood itself pouring back over one's finger. I could not help being impressed by the mechanical nature of these lesions and by the practicability of their surgical relief [1925, p. 606].

In spite of these heroic and unique accomplishments, further diagnostic and technical improvements were needed before the full potential of cardiac surgery could be realized. As far back as the mid-nineteenth century, French physiologists had positioned catheters or instruments in the hearts of animals for a variety of purposes. Claude Bernard (1813–1878) passed glass thermometers through the carotid artery into the left ventricle and through the jugular vein into the right heart chambers in order to determine where body heat originated. Using hollow glass tubes, he also measured pressure within the ventricular cavities (Comroe, 1983, p. 122). A few years later, Auguste Chauveau, a professor of veterinary medicine, and Étienne Jules Marey, a physician in Paris, made recordings of pressure levels within the heart of an experimental animal by introducing a long catheter with a double lumen through the jugular vein into the right side of the heart and by inserting a specially designed catheter into the left ventricle by way of the carotid artery (Cournand, 1964, pp. 49–50). Such procedures were, of course, at that time limited to use in physiology laboratories.

In 1912, Bleichroeder, Unger, and Loeb were reported to have passed catheters into veins and into the right side of the heart of a human subject, although without x-ray documentation (Litwak, 1971, pp. 17–18). The first radiologically confirmed placement of such a cardiac catheter in a human took place seventeen years later. Werner Forssmann, a registrar in the surgical department at Augusta-Viktoria Hospital in Eberswalde, near Berlin, explained that his experiences with cardiac emergencies "led me to seek a new route by which the heart can be safely penetrated, and thus I attempted the *catheterization of the right heart from the venous system*" (1929, p. 252). Forssmann inserted a ureteral catheter into his own arm vein, guided it toward the heart, and with an x-ray picture confirmed that the tip of the catheter was located within the right atrium. In addition to this experiment upon himself, the report by Forssmann also described the clinical use of this procedure in a patient with a severe circulatory condition secondary to a ruptured appendix and purulent peritonitis in whom a catheter was inserted through an arm vein for a distance of sixty centimeters. In spite of treatment with fluids and medications through the catheter, the patient died from the effects of the disease. At autopsy, the catheter was found "as was intended, extending from the cephalic vein down into the right atrium. From there it proceeded another 2 cm into the inferior vena cava. No changes in the vascular intima or the valves could be found, and there also was no thrombus formation" (1929, p. 254). Forssmann's report also outlined some of the technical advantages and possible therapeutic indications for using this procedure in humans (1929, pp. 254–255).

The cardiac catheterization procedure described by Forssmann was used by radiologists to perform angiocardiography in order to visualize the great blood-vessels and the chambers of the heart. Shortly thereafter, by applying the procedure of right heart catheterization in humans, Cournand and Ranges measured the oxygen and carbon dioxide content of blood within the right auricle (1941), using this information to determine cardiac output by the well-known Fick method (Hamilton and Richards, 1964, pp. 96–97). In addition, Richards, Cournand, Darling, Gillespie, and Baldwin demonstrated that pressures within this chamber of the heart could be accurately recorded in man by means of the catheter under both normal conditions and in the presence of right heart failure (1942). As techniques and equipment for performing both right and left heart catheterization improved in the years that followed, the diagnostic value of these procedures for determining the altered anatomic and pathophysiologic features of congenital cardiac malformations, valve lesions, conditions related to heart failure, and pulmonary disorders was increasingly recognized, directing physicians with greater confidence toward appropriate medical therapy and surgical interventions. For their remarkable achievements, the Nobel Prize for Medicine or Physiology was awarded to Forssmann, Cournand, and Richards in 1956.

During the 1930s, numerous surgical procedures were devised to increase the blood supply to the heart in order to relieve symptoms of angina. Claude Beck in the United States placed pedicle grafts of skeletal muscle around the heart, using pectoral muscles from the chest for this purpose (1935), while Laurence O'Shaughnessy in England performed cardio-omentopexy for a similar reason, applying richly vascularized omentum to the heart wall (1937). Many patients appeared to improve, suggesting that a collateral blood supply to the heart muscle had been created and that the heart had been revascularized. Modifications of these procedures followed, perhaps the best known of which was the technique proposed by Vineburg of Montreal. He stated that "The left internal mammary artery when transplanted into the wall of the left ventricle formed an anastomosis with the left coronary artery system after four months" (1946, p. 119). Many years later, F. Mason Sones, Jr., at the Cleveland Clinic confirmed with angiography that communications between the implanted artery and the coronary circulation were indeed present (Litwak, 1971, pp. 38–39), convincing skeptics that surgery to improve the heart's blood supply was a rational approach.

As these events were taking place, other investigators were carefully defining the complex cardiovascular anatomical changes in patients with congenital diseases. The painstaking work of Maud Abbott (1936) and of Helen Taussig (1947) made it apparent that if a precise diagnosis could be made, surgery might be able to correct many of these defects. Indeed, in a paper read before the Philadelphia Academy of Surgery many years earlier, John Munro had previously discussed the technical possibility of ligating a patent ductus arteriosus, a communication between the aorta and pulmonary artery that persists after birth, stating that

> long ago I demonstrated its technical possibility [ligation of a patent ductus arteriosus] on the cadaver of newborn children, and felt that it was justifiable on the living. At various times I have tried to inspire the pediatric specialist with my views, but in vain. Now, in view of recent advances in cardiac surgery . . . I will venture to place my ideas before you, asking that you do not dismiss them hastily [1907, p. 335].

Thirty-two years were to elapse following Munro's presentation before Gross and Hubbard at Boston's Children's Hospital described the successful ligation of a patent ductus arteriosus in a seven-year-old girl (1939). A few years later, the attention of the world was drawn to the miraculous results of the "blue-baby" operation, presented in a

memorable and dramatic report by Blalock and Taussig that concluded
with this summary:

> An operation for increasing the flow of blood through the lungs and
> thereby reducing the cyanosis in patients with congenital malformations of the
> heart consists in making an anastomosis between a branch of the aorta and one
> of the pulmonary arteries; in other words, the creation of an artificial ductus
> arteriosus. Thus far the procedure has been carried out on only 3 children,
> each of whom had a severe degree of anoxemia. Clinical evidence of improve-
> ment has been striking and includes a pronounced decrease in the intensity
> of the cyanosis, a decrease in dyspnea and an increase in tolerance to exercise.
> In the 2 cases in which such laboratory studies were performed there has been
> a decline in the red blood cell count, in the hemoglobin and in the hematocrit
> reading, an increase in the oxygen content of the arterial blood, a fall in the
> oxygen capacity, and most significantly a decided rise in the oxygen saturation
> of the arterial blood.
> The types of abnormalities which should be benefited by this operation
> are the tetralogy of Fallot, pulmonary atresia with or without dextroposition
> of the aorta and with or without defective development of the right ventricle,
> a truncus arteriosus with bronchial arteries, and a single ventricle with a ru-
> dimentary outlet chamber in which the pulmonary artery is diminutive in size.
> The operation is indicated only when there is clinical and radiologic evidence
> of a decrease in the pulmonary blood flow. The operation is not indicated in
> cases of complete transposition of the great vessels or in the so-called "tetralogy
> of Fallot of the Eisenmenger type," and probably not in aortic atresia. It must
> be emphasized that the operation should not be performed when studies reveal
> a prominent pulmonary conus or pulsations at the hili of the lungs [1945, p.
> 202].

After World War II, surgeons were able to turn in earnest from
the area of trauma surgery and war injuries to the field of heart surgery.
Within the span of a few years, operative procedures on the mitral
valve that had been devised in the 1920s by Cutler and Levine (1923)
and by Souttar (1925) were improved upon by Harken, Ellis, Ware,
and Norman in Boston (1948), by Bailey in Philadelphia (1949), and
by Baker, Brock, and Campbell in England (1950). Closed mitral valve
surgery rapidly became a reality. However, it was not long before the
limitations of this form of heart surgery and the potential advantages
and broader opportunities of open-heart procedures became evident,
particularly for valve replacement and correction of complex congenital
heart malformations. Although direct-vision cardiac surgery could be
successfully accomplished using hypothermic techniques to lower body
temperature and reduce total body oxygen consumption, thus giving
surgeons additional time to operate (Bigelow, Lindsay, and Greenwood, 1950), the era of open-heart surgery had to await the monu-

mental work of John Gibbon, Jr., of Philadelphia. During the 1930s and 1940s, Gibbon had been working on a heart-lung machine, which he described as follows:

> An apparatus which embodies a mechanical lung, as well as pumps, enables you to shunt blood around both the heart and lungs, thus allowing operations to be performed under direct vision in a bloodless field within the opened heart. Furthermore, an apparatus which embodies a mechanical lung enables you to provide partial support to either a failing heart or failing lung where a major operative procedure is not contemplated. Such an apparatus can also be used as an adjunct during the course of a major operative procedure. This partial support of the cardiorespiratory functions consists in removing venous blood from some peripheral vein continuously, oxygenating the blood and getting rid of the carbon dioxide in it and then injecting the blood continuously in a central direction in a peripheral artery. Of course, such partial circulation, or cardiorespiratory support, requires the use of a mechanical lung in the circuit [1954, p. 171].

On May 6, 1953, Gibbon repaired a large atrial septal defect in an eighteen-year-old girl while "for twenty-six minutes all cardiorespiratory functions were maintained by the apparatus [the heart-lung machine]" (1954, p. 176). As so eloquently expressed by Leo Eloesser, cardiac surgery had received its most powerful tool:

> Gibbon's idea and its elaboration take their place among the boldest and most sucessful [sic] feats of man's mind—with invention of the phonetic alphabet, the telephone, or a Mozartian symphony. Not a Deus ex machina but a machina a Deo; a Promethean fire; leveling from God His secrets to man's understanding; the pulse of the sacred heart; the breath of life [1970, p. 162].

At this point, the field of cardiac surgery was inundated by a plethora of contributions, including pacemaker therapy, repair of more complex congenital cardiac malformations, implantation of prosthetic heart valves, coronary artery bypass graft procedures, and the awe-inspiring achievements of heart transplantation and the artificial heart—all notable accomplishments of more recent origin. If past form holds true, further progress will be limited only by the skill and imagination of those involved.

26

Cardiac Pacing: Its Formative Years

For many years before cardiac pacing became a clinical reality, the effects of electrical stimulation of the heart had intrigued scientists, medical practitioners, and the public alike. The ability to produce electricity with the Leyden jar and with the electric cell of Alessandro Volta gave investigators an opportunity to study this phenomenon experimentally. At the turn of the nineteenth century, "an amazingly zealous researcher" named Nysten (Schechter, 1971b, pp. 2576–2578) described the variable responsiveness of different parts of the heart to electrical stimulation after death, his studies performed on at least one occasion in the freshly dug grave of a newly executed criminal. A few years later, John Aldini wrote in his work, *General Views on The Application of Galvanism to Medical Purposes: Principally in cases of suspended animation:*

> The before-mentioned Professors have, by these three procedures observed on many decapitated persons strong contractions of the heart, and have ascertained that the apex is of all its parts the most susceptible of motion, and of galvanic power. They observed also that, next to the intestines, the heart was the first to lose its susceptibility to galvanism [Schechter, p. 2578].

Thus, it was demonstrated that the ability of different parts of the heart to respond to electrical stimulation after death varied, and that such responsiveness persisted only for a limited time. The relevance and significance of these findings, although obtained by crudely performed studies, can be appreciated when examined in the light of subsequent developments in cardiac pacemaker therapy.

Perhaps one of the most unusual descriptions of the effects of electricity upon the heart of a live human being was reported in 1882 in the German medical literature by Hugo von Ziemssen, professor of medicine at Munich. Following removal of a tumor, an enchondroma, a forty-two-year-old woman named Catharina Serafin was left with a huge defect of the left side of her chest exposing the heart. In a manner reminiscent of William Beaumont's classic and well-known observations of the exposed lining of the stomach in a patient with a gunshot wound of the abdomen (Beaumont, 1833), von Ziemssen similarly seized the opportunity to study the heart, placing electrodes within the area of the chest wound or directly on the beating heart and noting the influence of voltaic currents of various intensities and frequencies upon the pulse rate. According to Schechter, as a result of these experiments, he, von Ziemssen, was "induced . . . to try the effect of the voltaic current in persons with the thorax intact. . . . [H]e arrived at the conclusion that it was possible to modify at will the action of the heart by means of currents of sufficient intensity and frequency" (1972a, p. 398).

Although many investigators made significant contributions to the field of cardiac electrical stimulation and electro-physiology during the late nineteenth century, the following excerpts from the work of John McWilliam at the University of Aberdeen are selected as a particularly revealing example of the keen insight and imagination demonstrated by these early pioneers, many times working as they did in an environment that would be considered rudimentary by today's standards:

> We want a much more effective and speedy mode of exciting rhythmic contraction, and one that will have a direct and powerful influence in calling forth a series of beats in the depressed or inhibited heart, while at the same time free from the danger of throwing the ventricles into delirium [ventricular fibrillation]. Such a mode of excitation seems to be available in the form of a periodic series of single induction shocks sent through the heart at approximately the normal rate of cardiac action. A single induction shock readily causes a beat in an inhibited heart, and a regular series of induction shocks (for example, sixty or seventy per minute) gives a regular series of heartbeats at the same rate [1889, p. 349].

Using an anesthetized animal, McWilliam described how he slowed the heart

> by stimulation of the vagus nerve in the neck, and then a periodic series of induction shocks (regulated by a metronome) was applied to the apex of the

ventricles. Contraction of the auricles and ventricles was recorded by an ad-
aptation of the graphic method; a blood-pressure tracing was simultaneously
made in the usual manner. In this way I was able to obtain an accurate record
of the various changes, while at the same time some further information was
obtained by direct inspection of the heart. A series of single induction shocks
excites a corresponding series of cardiac beats; the ventricular contraction pre-
cedes the auricular contraction when the exciting shocks are applied to the
ventricles. Each systole causes the ejection of a considerable amount of blood
into the aorta and pulmonary artery, and a marked rise of the blood-pressure
at each beat [1889, p. 349].

McWilliam concluded: "Such a method, it seems to me, is the
only rational and effective one for stimulating by direct means the
action of a heart which has been suddenly enfeebled or arrested in
diastole by causes of a temporary and transient character" (1889, p.
350).

The remarkable quality of the work done by von Ziemssen and
McWilliam during the latter years of the nineteenth century becomes
clear when it is recalled that more than another half a century elapsed
before Paul Zoll (1952) translated these observations into clinical usefulness for the treatment of ventricular standstill by external electrical
stimulation.

As far back as the early 1900s, investigators were placing catheter
electrodes into animals in order to stimulate the inner surface of the
heart, the endocardium, without having to perform open chest surgery
(Schechter, 1972b). In 1905, Floresco passed a glass sound through
the external jugular vein into the right ventricle. Copper or platinum
wires were introduced through the tube, and by means of induction
currents the endocardial surface of the heart was excited. Using a
similar technique to examine the endocardial lining of the heart chambers, Marmorstein in 1927 defined regional differences in the heart's
response to electrical excitation (Schechter, 1972b, pp. 608–609).
Another thirty years were to pass before this procedure was used for
intracardiac pacing in patients with heart block (Furman and Robinson, 1958; Furman and Schwedel, 1959).

A milestone in cardiac pacing was achieved in the early 1930s
when Albert Hyman in New York demonstrated experimentally that
a needle electrode placed into the heart and attached to an external
electrical power source could serve as an artificial pacemaker during
cardiac standstill (Hyman, 1932). The relevance and significance of
this important work are best conveyed by Hyman's summary:

3. In using a clinical needle through which is carried an electric impulse, and in having the two electrodes so close together that only a small pathway is concerned in the electric arc established by the heart muscle, an irritable point is produced.

4. This irritable point becomes the focus from which an excitation wave may spread over the heart muscle, the excitation wave developing and spreading according to normal physiologic conditions. The impulse released from the pacemaker needle differs in no way from that produced by the prick of any injecting needle except that in the latter instance only one stimulus is developed, while in the former any number can be delivered to the heart muscle.

5. An apparatus has been constructed which attempts to simulate the excitation wave developed by the normal sinus nodal pacemaker; it consists in a special current generated by a magneto which is activated by a spring motor, making it instantaneously available at any time, at any place and under all circumstances, as it is an independent electric unit. The current from this generator can be so regulated that the impulses are delivered to the needle point at a constant regular rate varying from 30 to 120 beats per minute. . . .

7. Experimental animal studies have shown that the arrested heart is rapidly returned to automatic sinus activity after the response to the artificial pacemaker has restored some of the normal circulatory balance. . . .

10. In view of the possible advantageous results to be anticipated by the use of the artificial pacemaker in the arrested heart which does not respond to the usual methods of therapy, the employment of this method is suggested. When patients have succumbed to disease processes, an attempt can be made to renew automatic cardiac activity by the use of the artificial pacemaker without in any way jeopardizing their condition.

11. When correctly used, the artificial pacemaker may prove to be of inestimable value in the restoration of those patients now succumbing to cardiac arrest; employed together with other established life-saving procedures it may well be included in every physician's armamentarium against the final struggle with death [1932, pp. 304–305].

Although a remarkable breakthrough, the time was not yet right for clinical application of this new technology. In part this may have been related to the need for a method of placing electrodes less drastic than directly inserting them through the chest wall, a somewhat awesome procedure and at best a temporary measure. In addition, further physician education and acceptance of pacemaker therapy was needed, as witness an amusing letter appearing in a medical journal requesting "information concerning the heart tickler" (Clauser, 1933).

During the 1950s and early 1960s, several significant studies took place that provided the framework for present-day pacemaker therapy. A landmark article entitled "Resuscitation of the heart in ventricular standstill by external electric stimulation" was published by Paul Zoll of the Harvard Medical School and Beth Israel Hospital in Boston describing "a quick, simple, effective and safe method of arousing the heart from ventricular standstill by an artificial, external, electric pace-maker. For the first time it was possible to keep a patient alive during ventricular asystole lasting for hours to days" (1952, p. 768). Further on in the text, Zoll continued: "Effective ventricular beats were reg-ularly produced in 2 patients with ventricular standstill after complete heart block by the application of electric stimuli from an artificial, external pacemaker by way of subcutaneous needle electrodes" (1952, p. 771). Zoll, Linenthal, and Norman (1954) expanded upon this experience in describing external cardiac pacemaker therapy for four-teen patients with Stokes-Adams disease.

One of the serious complications that may occur following surgery for complex congenital heart defects is the development of complete atrioventricular block. In an effort to manage this problem and main-tain patients until their own normal heart rhythms reappeared, Weir-ich, Gott, and Lillehei (1957) placed an insulated wire electrode in the wall of the heart at the time of surgery and attached it to an external pacemaker. Once heart block or the potential for heart block was no longer a threat and the pacemaker no longer needed, the wire could be removed without difficulty. Within the next few years, Chardack, Gage, and Greatbatch (1960) and Zoll, Frank, Zarsky, Linenthal, and Belgard (1961) in the United States, and Elmqvist, Landegren, Pet-tersson, Senning, and William-Olsson (1963) in Sweden extended this procedure to other patients with heart block by placing an electrode on the heart wall via a thoracotomy and attaching the electrode wire to a small battery-operated pulse generator implanted beneath the skin. The opportunities presented by the development of self-contained im-plantable pacemakers broadened the clinical scope of pacemaker ther-apy beyond its use as a temporary form of treatment and greatly reduced the inconvenience to patients who heretofore were tethered to a cum-bersome external device as a power source.

An electrical artificial pacemaker was used by Callaghan and Bigelow at the University of Toronto to stimulate heart action in animals during prolonged periods of experimentally produced cardiac arrest. The pacemaker electrode was inserted through a vein and po-sitioned at the site of the sino-auricular node:

> To approach the pacemaker without opening the chest an electrode of the two-point type was made up in a tube the size of a No. 12 French hard rubber venous catheter. The electrode was inserted into the right external jugular vein, passed through the superior vena cava until the stimulating tip lay in intimate

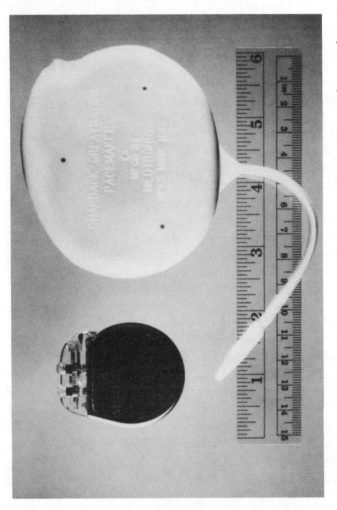

FIG. 26.1. Reflecting improved integrated circuitry and battery technology, the size of pacemakers implanted in the body has been markedly reduced during the last 2–3 decades. An early pacemaker from 1962, pictured on the right, measures 3¼ inches high, 3½ inches wide, and 1 inch thick. In contrast, a comparable pacemaker from 1989, shown on the left, is 2 inches high, 1⅝ inches wide, and only ¼ inch thick. *Source:* Courtesy of Medtronic Inc., Minneapolis, MN.

contact with the deep surface of the sino-auricular node at the junction of the superior vena cava and right atrium [Callaghan and Bigelow, 1951, p. 10].

Seven years later, Furman and Robinson (1958) outlined a similar procedure for passing an electrode catheter into the cavity of the right ventricle of dogs in order to stimulate the ventricle to contract by applying a low-voltage current directly to the endocardium. The following year, this technique was used (Furman and Schwedel, 1959) in treating two patients with Stokes-Adams seizures, thus providing physicians with the ability to perform transvenous pacing rapidly and safely without having to do a thoracotomy to implant the electrodes in the heart. The painful chest wall contractions experienced with external pacing were also able to be avoided. Shortly thereafter, this procedure was adapted for use as a permanent implantable pacemaker system (Parsonnet, Zucker, and Asa, 1962).

The basic concepts and techniques necessary for cardiac pacing were in place. Clinical indications for pacemaker therapy could now be expanded as further improvements and refinements were made in the design and performance of newer electrodes and pulse generators (Figure 26.1). Much had been accomplished since the days of "the heart tickler" (Clauser, 1933).

27

Prosthetic Heart Valves: A Tribute to Surgeons and Engineers

THE confluence of many new ideas within a short time enabled cardiac surgeons to enlarge the scope of their surgery and to turn from closed or nonvisual operations on damaged heart valves to open and direct visual methods for repairing and actually replacing the valves themselves. The use of cardiac catheterization in patients with diseased heart valves improved the physician's ability to assess preoperatively the severity of the hemodynamic impairment and permitted a suitable decision to be made regarding the potential benefits of surgery. In addition, heart-lung bypass, developed by John Gibbon during the 1930s and 1940s and culminating in the first clinical use of a heart-lung machine in the early 1950s (Gibbon, 1954), gave surgeons time to operate under direct vision within the heart itself. Still required, however, were suitable materials with which to construct functional and durable heart valves.

On the basis of experimental work during the 1940s, Charles Hufnagel at Georgetown University "demonstrated that materials properly shaped, having the characteristic of being well tolerated by tissue, having adequate strength, and high resistance to wetting could be used to successfully and permanently replace portions of the thoracic aorta" (1951, p. 128). Hufnagel showed that certain plastic materials such as methyl methacrylate had these characteristics, and that when shaped into a tube or valve could be placed in the ascending aorta of animals without the occurrence of thrombosis or disruption of the prosthesis. Since cardiopulmonary bypass was not yet a clinical reality at the time of this work, it was technically not possible to replace a patient's

195

diseased valve directly with a valve prosthesis. For the moment, therefore, placement of such an artificial valve was limited to positioning it in the aorta for treatment of aortic insufficiency, leaving the patient's own valve in place. After further experimentation and preparation, Hufnagel and Harvey were able to announce the following:

> A valve has now been designed suitable for application to clinical cases of aortic insufficiency. This is a ball-type valve similar to those used in the animal experiments. Already it has been considerably modified because of the increased mass of the ball necessitated by the large sizes of the valves employed. The ball which opens and closes to permit flow of blood during systole and prevents its backflow during diastole is of hollow "Plexiglas" [a plastic material], and the two halves of the ball are fused in such a way that the continuity of the surface is unbroken by any seam or roughness. The chamber for the ball is made of a single piece of "Plexiglas." These valves have been made in sizes of ¾", ⅞", 1" and 1⅛" to accommodate the varying aortic measurements which might be encountered in patients [1953, p. 60].

On September 11, 1952, the first person to receive the prosthetic ball valve was operated upon, a woman with severe aortic regurgitation and congestive heart failure (Hufnagel and Harvey, 1953). Within two years, the operation was successfully performed in several additional patients (Hufnagel, Harvey, Rabil, and McDermott, 1954). Hufnagel was later to remark on the significance of this historic procedure:

> The first successful clinical implantation of a ball valve in 1952 marked the introduction of the concept that it is possible to introduce into the cardio-vascular system a completely nonbiologic valvular device which could be activated by those forces generated by the heart itself and which could function satisfactorily within the vascular system for a relatively unlimited time [1979, p. 289].

It was noted that the sounds produced by the opening and closing of the first prosthetic valve implants could be heard not only by the patients themselves but also by those around them: "Proximity of the valve to the left main-stem bronchus always makes the valve audible if one listens to the patient who has the mouth open in a very quiet room (Hufnagel et al., 1954, p. 682). Several years later, in their well-known book, *Clinical Auscultation of the Heart*, Levine and Harvey related some amusing anecdotes about the clicking sounds produced by the ball component of this valve as it was thrust back and forth during systole and diastole, striking the ends of the chamber in which it was contained:

> Initially, we were concerned that the noise produced by the valve might be a most distracting symptom. In fact, the first patient who received the plastic artificial aortic valve had loud clicking sounds coming from her chest. These were easily heard with the naked ear. Purposely, for approximately two weeks postoperatively, no one discussed the sound of the valve with the patient. Finally she was asked if these sounds bothered her. After some deliberation the patient remarked, "No, they don't bother me, but it would bother me if I didn't hear them." Another patient stated that he personally did not mind the clicking sounds and paid no attention to them, except when playing poker. Every time he got a good hand the sounds became louder because of his excitement, thereby giving away his secret to his fellow players [1959, p. 306].

In later models, the design and material of the ball were changed to a hollow nylon core coated with highly compressed, heat-cured silicone rubber, markedly reducing disturbing sounds (Hufnagel, 1979, p. 289).

With the experience gained from Hufnagel's experiments, and with the advantages gained from using open heart techniques, other approaches to the problems of valve replacement were undertaken. The failure of operative procedures that attempted a direct repair of a diseased valve had prompted Harken, Soroff, Taylor, Lefemine, Gupta, and Lunzer in Boston to evaluate

> the construction of a complete valve. In view of difficulties with fatigue studies, we sought materials that have been tested, namely, the Lucite balls of the Hufnagel valve, or preferably the more recent, quiet, silicone rubber-covered ball. These have been in place in human beings since 1955.
>
> A stainless steel caged-ball valve has been built. The orifice is 1.98 sq. cm. The inner cage must allow the ball to move far enough away from the base so that it does not obstruct flow, but if it is too long the ball can move so far away that there may be delay in return and, thus, reflux. The inner cage is of close tolerance for rapid seating [1960, p. 748].

Harken et al. successfully replaced a diseased aortic valve with this caged-ball prosthetic valve, noting at the conclusion of their report that "Special recognition and appreciation are due Mr. W. Clifford Birtwell, Chief Research Engineer of the Davol Company, for his remarkable ability to design and produce these valves and testing equipment" (1960, p. 761).

With prosthetic valve surgery now a viable option, it was even more urgent not only to plan for the best possible surgical procedure, anesthetic care, and pre- and postoperative management of patients, but also to work closely with engineers and other scientists in constructing valves that were durable, functional, efficient, noiseless, and sterilizeable, that would cause no foreign-body reaction or damage to blood, and that would not be a source of blood clots. Such collaborative activities led to a greater understanding of the intricacies of valve function, to a better appreciation of blood coagulation problems and material biocompatibility, and to the development of pulse duplicators that, by replicating the hemodynamic and physiological features of the cardiac cycle, allowed the competence of experimental valves to be evaluated. Many years later, these early observations were to have considerable relevance in the evolution of other prosthetic devices, particularly in the development of the artificial heart.

Following these pioneering efforts of the team at Georgetown University Medical Center led by Hufnagel and of the group headed by Harken in Boston, the next major accomplishment in valve design and implantation took place at the University of Oregon through the combined efforts of a surgeon, Albert Starr, and an engineer, Lowell Edwards. After testing a variety of valve prototypes and operative procedures in animals, a ball-valve prosthesis was designed for insertion into humans:

> The case is cast in one piece stainless steel or Satellite 21 and the final dimensions are achieved from the crude castings by machining or grinding. A mirror finish is produced by buffing and electro-polishing. The surface is then silicone coated and carefully inspected. Unless flawless with regard to minor imperfections or irregularities of surface the valve is rejected from further assembly. The knitted Teflon cloth fixation ring is attached by Teflon spreader rings and braided Teflon thread. The ball is of Dow-Corning medical grade heat-cured silastic [Starr and Edwards, 1961, p. 726].

The resources of companies such as Dow-Corning, U.S. Catheter and Instrument Company, and Precision Metalsmiths Incorporated contributed significantly to the development of this valve, reinforcing the proposition that benefits were to be derived from a close association between medicine and industry. With the implantation of this valve into the hearts of eight patients to replace diseased mitral valves (Starr and Edwards, 1961), another major step toward making valve replacement surgery a feasible procedure had occurred (Figure 27.1).

Despite experience with aortic valve allografts (valves obtained at postmortem examination) and pulmonary valve autografts (the patient's own tissue) to replace diseased valves, the emphasis appeared to be on developing other types of prostheses. Thus, a variety of new mechanical and tissue valves appeared, each model attempting to maximize du-

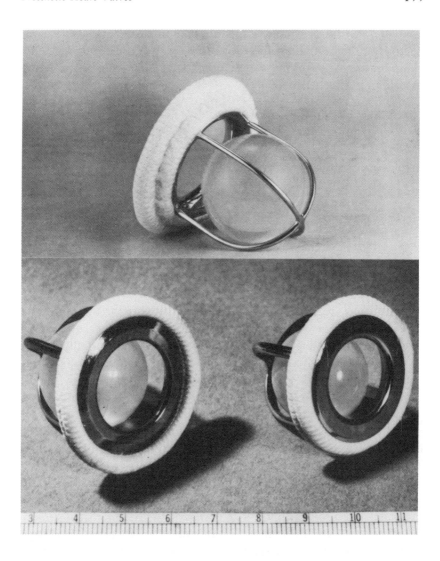

FIG. 27.1. Early models of Starr-Edwards prosthetic heart valves. The bottom picture shows a view of the inlet side of a pre-6000 mitral caged-ball prosthesis, available 1960–1964, with four stellite struts joined at the apex, a double donut valve base, a radiolucent poppet (ball) within the cage, and a woven sewing ring. The top photograph shows the outlet side of a later model 6000 mitral caged-ball prosthesis, available in 1964–1965, with four stellite struts meeting at the apex, a radiolucent poppet, and a cloth sewing ring. *Source:* Courtesy of Baxter Healthcare Corporation, Edwards CVS Division.

rability, to minimize the risk of thromboembolism, and to improve hemodynamic function still further. Harken and Curtis outlined a list of ten requirements (commandments?) that would be necessary for the success of a prosthetic valve:

1. It must not propagate emboli.
2. It must be chemically inert and not damage blood elements.
3. It must offer no resistance to physiologic flows.
4. It must close promptly (less than 0.05 sec.).
5. It must remain closed during the appropriate phase of the cardiac cycle.
6. It must have lasting physical and geometric features.
7. It must be inserted in a physiologic site, generally the normal anatomic site.
8. It must be capable of permanent fixation.
9. It must not annoy the patient.
10. It must be technically practical to insert [1967, p. 400].

Tilting disc valves, caged disc valves, bileaflet valves, ball-in-cage valves, and tissue prostheses prepared from pig valves, fascia lata, or pericardium were developed in an attempt to achieve these and possibly other requirements necessary for satisfactory performance of a valve. Each new valve had its enthusiastic proponents and was usually known by the name(s) of the inventor(s) or institution involved in its development, e.g., Bjørk-Shiley, Lillehei-Kaster, Ionescu-Shiley, Hancock, Carpentier-Edwards, St. Jude Medical (Black, Drury, and Tindale, 1983).

Although valve surgery has been life-saving and has permitted many patients to lead fruitful lives, the diversity of prosthetic devices available suggests that none has been entirely satisfactory in matching the wonders of nature's own remarkable creation. Thus, even while present valves continue to be improved, it should be a constant goal to reduce and insofar as possible to eliminate the need for such surgery by focusing on the prevention of valve diseases. Programs that have been under way for many years for preventing and treating rheumatic fever and other causes of valve damage, involving many different medical disciplines, are steps in the right direction.

28

Heart Transplantation: From Fantasy to Reality

> The human heart has hidden treasures,
> In secret kept, in silence sealed.
> [Brontë, 1846, p. 58]

ALTHOUGH successful human organ transplantation, particularly heart transplantation, has become a reality only in recent memory, the interchange of parts of human and animal bodies has long exerted fascination—e.g., as evidenced in mythological references to the centaur and the sphinx in ancient Greek and Egyptian times. In the introduction to *Huang Ti Nei Ching Su Wên—The Yellow Emperor's Classic of Internal Medicine*, Veith refers to a famous Chinese surgeon of the second century B.C. named Pien Ch'iao, who was said to have exchanged the hearts of two patients (1949, p. 3), while a well-known legend from Western culture relates how Cosmas and Damian of the third century A.D., the patron saints of doctors, transplanted the leg of a dead person to a patient whose own limb had been amputated (Dewhurst, 1988). Such tales aside, early grafting and transplantation experiments were performed by the nineteenth-century English surgeon John Hunter, who transplanted a human tooth into the vascular comb of a cock, and by Charles-Edouard Brown-Séquard (1817–1894), who, in spite of all his other well-known work, is sometimes best remembered for having injected testicular extracts into animals and

201

humans, including himself, in order "to rejuvenate his own waning powers" (Saunders, 1972, p. 16).

The first serious attempt at experimental heart transplantation has been credited to the Frenchman and 1912 Nobel prize recipient Alexis Carrel and to his colleague Charles Guthrie, an American physiologist, who, working together at the University of Chicago on experimental blood vessel surgery and reimplantation, wrote:

> The heart of a small dog was extirpated and transplanted into the neck of a larger one by anastomosing the cut ends of the jugular vein and the carotid artery to the aorta, the pulmonary artery, one of the vena cava and a pulmonary vein. The circulation was reestablished through the heart, about an hour and 15 minutes after the cessation of the beat; 20 minutes after the reestablishment of the circulation, the blood was actively circulating through the coronary system. A small opening being made through the wall of a small branch of the coronary vein, an abundant dark hemorrhage was produced. Then strong fibrillar contractions were seen. Afterward contractions of the auricles appeared, and, about an hour after the operation, effective contractions of the ventricles began. The transplanted heart beat at the rate of 88 per minute, while the rate of the normal heart was 100 per minute. A little later, tracings were taken. Owing to the fact that the operation was made without aseptic technic, coagulation occurred in the cavities of the heart after about two hours, and the experiment was interrupted [Carrel and Guthrie, 1905, pp. 1101–1102].

It was twenty-eight years later before the next significant report on cardiac transplantation appeared. Mann, Priestly, Markowitz, and Yater described a technique for transplanting a heart into the neck of a dog, with the donor animal's aorta anastomosed to the recipient's carotid artery, and the donor's pulmonary artery attached to the recipient's jugular vein. The operation provided for perfusion of the donor heart, referred to as "viviperfusion" (1933, p. 224), allowing the investigators to comment "that the transplanted heart should be a valuable test object for the investigation of various physiologic problems" (p. 224). The average survival time of a heart transplanted in this manner was four days. When removed and examined, "The surface of the [transplanted] heart was covered with mottled areas of ecchymosis; the heart was friable on section. Histologically the heart was completely infiltrated with lymphocytes, large mononuclears and polymorphonuclears" (p. 223). On the basis of these observations, the authors stated that "the failure of the homotransplanted heart to survive is not due to the technic of transplantation but to some biologic factor which is probably identical to that which prevents survival of other homotransplanted tissues and organs" (p. 224).

Thus, the problem of graft rejection of the transplanted heart was recognized. Several years later, experimental heart transplants were performed by Marcus, Wong, and Luisada "with the anastomoses so arranged that the left heart, as well as the right heart, is a functioning organ. To accomplish this an arterial supply from the host was anastomosed to a pulmonary vein of the heart transplant and an outlet for the left ventricular output of the heart transplant was provided" (1951, p. 217). Concern about the rejection phenomenon was still paramount, however, with the comment being made that "the greatest deterrent to long survival of the transplanted heart is the biologic problem of tissue specificity involved in any homologous transplantation" (1951, p. 216). The authors speculated that the idea of using a transplanted heart or heart-lung preparation as a replacement for a diseased organ "must be considered, at present [1951], a fantastic dream" (p. 216).

For the most part, transplant surgery had so far focused on the use of donor hearts as accessory organs or auxiliary pumps. In 1955, Demikhov in the Soviet Union, without operative support from a heart-lung machine or from hypothermic techniques, replaced the hearts of two animals, with postoperative survival provided solely by the activity of the transplanted hearts for 11½ and 15½ hours, respectively (Cooper, 1984, pp. 6–7). Five years later, in recipient animals prepared for circulatory bypass with a rotating disc oxygenator, Lower and Shumway at Stanford University School of Medicine were able to extend the survival time following transplantation of a donor heart, with five animals living for 6 to 21 days. During convalescence from the surgery, the transplanted denervated hearts initially appeared to function normally. The terminal course was usually quick, with postmortem examination indicating that "the massive infiltration of round cells and interstitial hemorrhage produces rapid myocardial failure" (1960, p. 19). As so clearly stated by these investigators, "Observations on these animals suggest that, if the immunologic mechanisms of the host were prevented from destroying the graft, in all likelihood it would continue to function adequately for the normal life span of the animal" (p. 19).

Schwartz, Stack, and Damashek at Tufts University School of Medicine (1958) demonstrated that 6-mercaptopurine, an antagonist of nucleic acid metabolism, can suppress the antibody response to a purified antigen. By combining such therapy with corticosteroids on a daily schedule, physicians at Stanford were able to improve the mean survival time of animals receiving a heart transplant from 7 to 17 days (Lower, Dong, and Shumway, 1965). When treatment was given intermittently during periods of threatened rejection rather than con- tinuously, survival time in some animals was prolonged even further. Using a somewhat different approach—that of profound hypothermia —other investigators showed that prolonged survival could be obtained in puppies undergoing heart homotransplantation without immuno- suppressive therapy, with one animal surviving 112 days (Kondo, Grädel, and Kantrowitz, 1965). It was postulated that transplantation in an immature animal might result in acceptance of the grafted heart for a more extended period of time.

Aside from studies of immunologic problems and of different surgical techniques, experiments were also designed to evaluate the physiologic and metabolic effects of cardiac autotransplantation. By excising a heart and then reimplanting it in the same animal, such effects could be determined without the associated problems of graft rejection. Although the possibility was raised that there might be spe- cific adverse consequences due to severed lymphatic channels and neural pathways of the reimplanted heart (Willman, Cooper, Cian, and Hanlon, 1962), this was not felt to be a major problem by the Stanford group of investigators, who stated: "After two years, in 4 cardiac autotransplants, innervation has recurred and myocardial func- tion is essentially normal. These studies suggest that there will be little physiologic objection to cardiac transplantation" (Dong, Hurley, Lower, and Shumway, 1964, p. 273).

So far, investigations of cardiac transplantation had been limited to the animal laboratory. In a desperate attempt to save the life of an ill patient, a group from the University Hospital of the University of Mississippi Medical Center replaced a human heart with a heart from a 96-pound chimpanzee, a human donor heart not being available at the time (Hardy, Chavez, Kurrus, Neely, Eraslan, Turner, Fabian, and Labecki, 1964). The transplanted heart, with the aid of a pace- maker, maintained a blood pressure level ranging from 60 to 90 mm. Hg after the operation was completed. Unfortunately, the donor heart was unable to accommodate the large venous return, and the effort was discontinued after 1–2 hours. The authors concluded, however, that "this experience supports the scientific feasibility of heart transplantation in man" (1964, p. 1140).

Three years later, in December 1967, before a startled and fascinated world audience, Dr. Christiaan Barnard performed the first human-to-human heart transplant at Groote Schuur Hospital in Cape Town, South Africa. Acknowledging the vital efforts of his predecessors— "Steady progress towards this goal [human heart transplantation] has been made by immunologists, biochemists, surgeons and specialists in other branches of medical science all over the world during the past decades to ensure that this, the ultimate in cardiac surgery, would be a success" (1967, p. 1271)— Barnard replaced the diseased heart of a man in his mid-50s with one from a human donor. The recipient of the new heart, Louis Washkansky, survived 18 days, succumbing to pneumonia. A month later, Philip Blaiberg underwent a similar operation at the same hospital, subsequently leading a full life for over 1½ years as the first long-term survivor of heart transplant surgery (Barnard, 1968; Cooper and Lanza, 1984). What once had been fantasy was now reality.

In January 1968, the human cardiac transplant program began at Stanford University Medical Center under the pioneering and outstanding leadership of Norman Shumway. Nearly 13½ years later, this group presented its experience based upon 227 transplant procedures performed from the inception of the program to April, 1981 (Pennock, Oyer, Reitz, Jamieson, Bieber, Wallwork, Stinson, and Shumway, 1982). The proportion of patients surviving at one year after heart transplantation increased from 22 percent in 1968 to 67 percent in 1979, an encouraging result that reflected improved criteria for selection of recipients, the introduction of rabbit anti-human thymocyte globulin for immune suppression, and close postoperative observation for acute graft rejection by means of clinical electrocardiography, immunologic monitoring, and frequent right ventricular endomyocardial biopsies. The leading causes of early and late post-transplantation deaths were infection, acute rejection, graft arteriosclerosis, and malignancy, in decreasing order of frequency, with a 39 percent survival rate at five years after transplantation. Also discussed by these authors were the potential number of cardiac transplant recipients that might be anticipated in the future based upon the availability of suitable donors and the high costs of such a program, estimated at first-year costs of $130,000 per patient including transplant hospitalizations, follow-up hospitalizations, and outpatient visits. The authors concluded that "On the basis of this consideration and the survival and rehabilitation data presented, we believe that the cost of cardiac transplantation is justified in selected individuals" (Pennock et al., 1982, p. 176). For those whose enthusiasm may sometimes take precedence over good judgment, a thoughtful and cautionary reminder about the limits of cardiac transplantation was added by Pennock in the brief discussion at the conclusion of this paper: "Cardiac transplantation or mechanical heart replacement is not a realistic method by which to achieve immortality" (p. 177).

A recent addition to immunosuppressive drug therapy after heart transplantation is cyclosporin A, a preparation that Borel, Feurer, Gubler, and Stähelin (1976) found to have a strong selectivity of action "at an early stage of antigenic triggering of immunocompetent cells" (p. 475). Preliminary observations by the Stanford cardiac transplant team (Pennock et al., 1982, pp. 174–175) suggested that this drug decreased the incidence of lethal infections and rejection episodes in the early postoperative period and thus might be a useful addition to the immunologic armamentarium.

Although cardiac transplantation has currently become a reasonable and acceptable form of therapy, the procedure had provoked much discussion among scientists, bioethicists, legal experts, clergymen, and politicians. History will rightfully praise the marvel of this technologic achievement, although in the long run the ability of our generation to understand and to cope with the ethical, moral, social, and economic dilemmas associated with it may well have the more decisive influence upon its future role in medical practice.

29

Echocardiography: Echoes from the Heart

Blow, bugle, blow, set the wild echoes flying.
[Alfred Tennyson, 1847, p. 134]

F EIGENBAUM gave the following concise descriptions of echocardiography and of ultrasound in his well-known textbook *Echocardiography*:

> Echocardiography is a diagnostic procedure that utilizes ultrasound to visualize the heart in a non-invasive manner. . . .
> By definition, ultrasound is sound with a *frequency* greater than 20 thousand cycles per second, which means that it is above the audible range. Actually, frequencies in the range of millions of cycles per second are used for medical diagnostic purposes [1972, p. 5].

As noted by Wells (1978) in reviewing the history of ultrasound, the piezoelectric effect was detected in 1880 by Pierre and Jacques Curie. The word "piezoelectric" is formed by combining the Greek *piezein*, meaning to press, with the word "electric." Certain materials such as quartz possess the property of changing their shapes under the influence of an electric field, vibrating rapidly and producing ultrasound waves. The reverse also happens: that is, when a piezoelectric substance is struck with ultrasound, an electric impulse is produced. Such piezoelectric substances are the primary components of the transducers or probes used in diagnostic ultrasonic equipment.

208

Medical Techniques and Treatments

In the early years of the twentieth century, the French scientist Paul Langevin developed a quartz crystal for generating and transmitting ultrasonic waves through water (Feigenbaum, 1972; Wells, 1978). During World War I, this work had significant applications in the detection of underwater objects, such as submarines, and has subsequently been regarded as the forerunner of modern sonar (the word "sonar" is an acronym for sound navigation and ranging). Improvements in instrumentation were slow in being developed between World Wars I and II, although an ultrasonic method for detecting flaws in metal was described in 1929 by the Russian scientist Sokolov (Feigenbaum, 1972, p. 1). However, prompted by the needs of the military, ultrasound technology expanded during World War II, again primarily for the purpose of detecting submarines, accompanied by the use of another form of technology using echoes, that of radar, the detection of echoes of radio waves—radio detecting and ranging.

Following World War II, Floyd Firestone of the Departments of Physics and Engineering Research at the University of Michigan published a report describing the use of pulsed reflected ultrasound for detecting flaws within metals, work that was to stimulate considerable interest in diagnostic uses of ultrasound in medicine during the years ahead. Firestone began his report as follows: "The supersonic reflectoscope is an instrument for the measurement or non-destructive testing of solid parts for flaws, by sending supersonic sound waves into the part and observing reflections from the boundaries of the part or from flaws within it" (1946, p. 287).

Of additional interest, particularly as it demonstrates that the necessary engineering prerequisites for the diagnostic application of ultrasound in medicine were already available during the mid-1940s, is this brief description by Firestone explaining the principle of his instrument:

Fig. 1. Principle of the supersonic reflectoscope. A quartz crystal making contact with the work through a thin film of oil sends into the work a wave group consisting of just a few sound waves of short wave-length. This wave group is reflected from the side of the work most distant from the crystal, and upon striking the crystal generates in it a voltage whose time of arrival is indicated on a cathode-ray oscilloscope. The flaw is detected by the fact that it reflects a part of the wave group back to the crystal and this reflection arrives at the crystal *before* the reflection from the distant side of the work [1946, p. 287].

In the 1940s, initial attempts at applying ultrasound for medical diagnostic purposes used the so-called transmission method, a procedure described by Dussik, Dussik, and Wyt (1947). A beam of ultrasound rays was directed through the head of a patient, with the differential absorption of wave forms by the various structures within the skull creating different patterns as the beam emerged and was recorded on the opposite side. The results with this technique, however, were not satisfactory. Instead, more reliable information was obtained by the pulse-echo method, mentioned in discussing the work of Firestone (1946). By the late 1940s, three independent investigators, George Ludwig, Douglas Howry, and John Wild, using the experience acquired from sonar development during World War II and the knowledge gained from metal flaw detectors, were able "to demonstrate that as ultrasound waves were sent into the body, echoes would return to the same transducer by reflection from tissue interfaces of different density" (Holmes, 1980, p. 299). Of particular interest during these early developmental years was the technique used by Wild and Reid (1952) for detecting tumors, it having been observed that variations of the echo pattern might differentiate benign from malignant disease. The same authors also suggested use of the general term "echography" for the entire subject in which the reflection of ultrasonic wave forms are used to examine biological tissue, with the basic electronic machine called the "echograph," the applicator units or probes called "echoscopes," and the records called "echograms" (1956, p. 248).

Carl Hellmuth Hertz, a physicist, and Inge Edler, a cardiologist, while at the University of Lund in Sweden, are credited with being the first to use reflected ultrasound in the field of cardiology. The interesting, low-key story of the events leading up to their initial publication is contained in their reminiscences many years later (Hertz, 1973; Edler and Hertz, 1977). During a meeting between Edler and Hertz in the early 1950s, the question was raised as to whether the new ultrasonic tool available for detecting flaws in metals, the ultrasonic reflectoscope, might be helpful in examining patients with cardiac problems, particularly in evaluating diseases of the mitral valve, a subject of great interest to Dr. Edler. Aware that such an instrument had recently been acquired by the Tekniska Röntgencentralen, a company specializing in nondestructive material testing at the ship-building yards of nearby Malmö, Hertz traveled there to see if he could obtain echoes from his own heart with the use of this machine. As they later described it, "To his pleasant surprise, he [Hertz] obtained well-defined echoes on the CRT [cathode-ray-tube] screen moving synchronously with his heart beat when he directed the ultrasonic beam towards his heart" (Edler and Hertz, 1977, p. 353). Permission was obtained to use the reflectoscope for a weekend, at the end of which time Hertz and Edler were convinced that this diagnostic approach should be evaluated more carefully. Lacking the funds to purchase such an instrument, they arranged to borrow a reflectoscope through the efforts of a contact at the medical branch of the Siemens Company in Erlangen, Germany—and the rest is history.

In their premier article entitled "The use of ultrasonic reflectoscope for the continuous recording of the movements of heart walls," Edler and Hertz (1954) explained the difference between earlier work done by Keidel using transmitted ultrasound and their own reflected-sound-pulse procedure (Figure 29.1). Experiments were described, first studying the isolated heart to verify that blood-heart wall boundaries could be detected with reflected sound waves, and then examining the human heart *in vivo* to evaluate motion of the heart walls. Their results were summarized at the conclusion of this report:

> 1) It has been shown that it is possible to locate blood-heart wall boundaries by the supersonic reflectoscope method using frequencies of about 2.5 Mc.
>
> 2) The method was applied for the locating of heart walls on living human beings and continuous registration of movements of the heart walls was found possible.
>
> 3) Recordings are shown of the movements of the left ventricle wall in the normal and in the diseased heart. Further, movements of the left atrial wall in mitral stenosis were recorded [1954, p. 57].

The difficulty in correctly interpreting these initial tracings was noted many years later by Hertz, who, in reviewing the development of echocardiography, stated: "It was not until 1959 that Dr. Edler could prove by probing needles during autopsy that the echoes recorded by him must have been generated by the mitral valves themselves" (1973, p. 8). Until then, it had been mistakenly thought that the echoes portrayed in many of these early graphs originated from the wall of the heart.

In one of his earlier communications, Edler (1955) indicated that this newly described technique could be used to differentiate pure mitral stenosis from mitral regurgitation, to diagnosis thrombosis in the left atrium, and to detect pericardial effusion. Technologic and

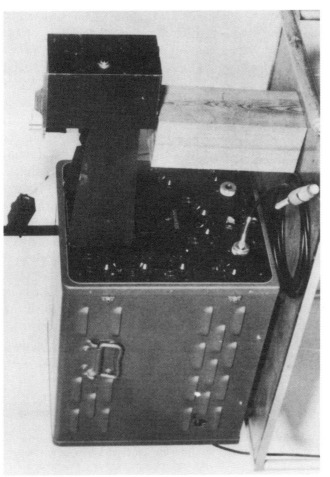

FIG. 29.1. The first echocardiography system used in clinical investigations during the early 1950s by Dr. Inge Edler and Professor C. Hellmuth Hertz at Lund University Hospital, Sweden. A camera is attached for registration of the M-mode recordings, with a lamp on top of the equipment to permit including the patient's electrocardiogram in the record. *Source:* With permission of Dr. Inge Edler and Professor C. Hellmuth Hertz, and of Siemens Medical Systems, Erlangen, Federal Republic of Germany.

engineering advances with more sensitive transducers using barium titanate or lead zirconate titanate as the piezoelectric element rather than quartz permitted better resolution of cardiac structures and more precise diagnosis. By designing equipment to meet the special demands of echocardiography, such early pioneers in this new field as Effert in Germany, and Joyner, Reid, Feigenbaum, and Gramiak in the United States, were able to explore additional applications. Diagnostic techniques and criteria were established for the clinical discipline of M-mode echocardiography, paving the way for a new generation of instruments and for the forthcoming appearance of two-dimensional echocardiography during the 1970s. In 1977, Edler and Hertz shared the prestigious Albert Lasker Award in Clinical Research for their contributions to this field.

The recently developed field of Doppler echocardiography utilizes the principle of the Doppler effect to obtain hemodynamic information, that is, the change in frequency of sound reflected from a column of blood as it moves with respect to the ultrasound transducer is used to calculate the blood's velocity and direction of flow within the cardiovascular system. With appropriate instrumentation and computations, pressure gradients, regurgitant flows, and shunt flows can be determined to assist in diagnosing the presence and severity of various disease states.

Doppler ultrasound techniques were named for Johann Christian Doppler, an Austrian mathematician and physicist who lived in the first half of the nineteenth century and described what came to be called the Doppler effect. His famous paper entitled "On the Coloured Light of Double Stars and Some other Heavenly Bodies," as summarized by White,

> begins by recapitulating the wave theory of light and explaining that the colour perceived by the eye varies with the frequency. He [Doppler] went on to postulate that this frequency will increase if the observer is moving towards the source and decrease if he is moving away from the source and drew an analogy of a ship moving to meet or retreat from a train of ocean waves [1982, p. 583].

Jonkman (1980) described an experiment performed by the Dutch scientist Buys Ballot during the mid-nineteenth century in which a musician-observer with perfect pitch perceived the sound of a horn on a moving locomotive as half a note higher approaching and half a note lower leaving the point of observation. With this and other similar experiments, the validity of Doppler's theoretical work with light was demonstrated and confirmed.

Since the publication of an article by Shigeo Satomura entitled "Ultrasonic Doppler method for the inspection of cardiac functions" (1957), interest and enthusiasm in Doppler echocardiography has expanded rapidly, with most current echocardiographic equipment now containing Doppler capabilities. Indeed, the appropriate use of this equipment can often provide important diagnostic and prognostic information without subjecting patients to the risks of invasive procedures such as angiography and cardiac catheterization.

The technologic achievements, widespread use, and successful application of ultrasound in cardiology represent the collaborative efforts of many disciplines working closely together, an important example of scientific teamwork, rightfully acknowledged and appreciated by Carl Hellmuth Hertz (1973) in his presentation at the 16th Annual Meeting of the American Institute of Ultrasound in Medicine entitled "The interaction of physicians, physicists and industry in the development of echocardiography."

Epilogue

By examining echoes as they are reflected from the heart of a patient, both a diagnosis and a reasonable assessment as to prognosis can be made. Similarly, by paying heed to echoes of past events, it may be possible not only to understand the present but in addition to plan and prepare for the future. It is hoped that the echoes reverberating in this book, aside from giving pleasure and enlightenment, can be put to such uses.

References

Abbott, M. E. (1936), *Atlas of Congenital Cardiac Disease*. New York: The American Heart Association.

Abel, J. J. (1926), Crystalline insulin. *Proc. Nat. Acad. Sci.*, 12:132–136.

——— Rowntree, L. G., & Turner, B. B. (1914), On the removal of diffusible substances from the circulating blood of living animals by dialysis. *J. Pharmacol. Exp. Ther.*, 5:275–316.

Addison, J., & Steele, R. (1709–1710), *The Tatler*, Vol. 3., No. 147. London: J. Richardson & Co., 1822, p. 199.

Addison, T. (1855), *On the Constitutional and Local Effects of Disease of the Suprarenal Capsules*. London: Samuel Highley.

Ahlquist, R. P. (1948), A study of the adrenotropic receptors. *Amer. J. Physiol.*, 153:586–600.

Allbutt, T. C. (1870), Medical thermometry. *Brit. & Foreign Med.-Chir. Rev.*, 45:429–441.

Allen, E. V., Barker, N. W., & Waugh, J. M. (1942), A preparation from spoiled sweet clover. *J. Amer. Med. Assn.*, 120:1009–1015.

Altshuler, I. M., & Shebesta, B. H. (1941), Music—An aid in management of the psychotic patient. *J. Nerv. & Ment. Dis.*, 94:179–183.

Annalen der Chemie und Pharmacie (1848), Editorial: Einwirkung der Mischung von Schwefelsäure und Salpetersäure auf einige organische Substanzen. *Annalen der Chemie und Pharmacie*, 64:396–398.

Arena, J. M. (1963), Atropine poisoning: A report of two cases from Jimson weed. *Clin. Pediat.*, 2:182–184.

Aretaeus, the Cappadocian (*c.* 120–200 A.D.), On the causes and symptoms of chronic diseases, Book 2, Ch. 2, On diabetes. In: *The Extant Works of Aretaeus, the Cappadocian*, ed. & trans. F. Adams. London: The Sydenham Society, 1856, pp. 338–340.

Aristotle (n.d.), History of animals. In: *Great Books of The Western World: The Works of Aristotle*, Vol. 2, trans. D'A. W. Thompson. Chicago, London, Toronto: William Benton Publisher, Encyclopaedia Britannica, Inc., 1952, pp. 7–158.

Arthus, M., & Pagès, C. (1890), Nouvelle théorie chimique de la coagulation du sang. *Arch. Physiol. norm. path.*, 2:739–746.

Auenbrugger, L. (1761), Inventum novum ex percussione thoracis humani, ut signo, abstrusos interni pectoris morbos detegendi [On Percussion of the Chest], trans. J. Forbes (1824). In: *Epoch-Making Contributions to Medicine, Surgery and the Allied Sciences*, ed. C. N. B. Camac. Philadelphia: W. B. Saunders Company, 1909, pp. 120–147.

Avicenna (n.d.), *A Treatise on the Canon of Medicine of Avicenna*, ed. O. C. Gruner. London: Luzac & Co., 1930.

Babylonian Talmud (n.d.a), *Seder Nezikin: Baba Bathra 1,58b*, ed. I. Epstein. London: The Soncino Press, 1935, p. 235.
────── (n.d.b), *Seder Zera'im: Berakoth, 35b*, ed. I. Epstein. London: The Soncino Press, 1948, p. 223.
Bailey, C. P. (1949), The surgical treatment of mitral stenosis (mitral commissurotomy). *Dis. Chest*, 15:377–397.
Baker, A. B. (1971), Artificial respiration, the history of an idea. *Med. Hist.*, 15:336–351.
Baker, C., Brock, R. C., & Campbell, M. (1950), Valvulotomy for mitral stenosis. *Brit. Med. J.*, 1:1283–1293.
Banting, F. G., & Best, C. H. (1922), The internal secretion of the pancreas. *J. Lab. Clin. Med.*, 7:251–266.
──────────── Collip, J. B., Campbell, W. R., & Fletcher, A. A. (1922), Pancreatic extracts in the treatment of diabetes mellitus. *Can. Med. Assn. J.*, 12:141–146.
Barcroft, J. (1920), Anoxaemia. *Lancet*, 2:485–489.
────── Cooke, A., Hartridge, H., Parsons, T. R., & Parsons, W. (1920), The flow of oxygen through the pulmonary epithelium. *J. Physiol.*, 53:450–472.
Barnard, C. N. (1967), A human cardiac transplant: An interim report of a successful operation performed at Groote Schuur Hospital, Cape Town. *S. Afr. Med. J.*, 41:1271–1274.
────── (1968), Human cardiac transplantation: An evaluation of the first two operations performed at the Groote Schuur Hospital, Cape Town. *Amer. J. Cardiol.*, 22:584–596.
Bartholow, R. (1882), *A Practical Treatise on Materia Medica and Therapeutics*. New York: D. Appleton & Co.
Beaumont, W. (1833), *Experiments and Observations on the Gastric Juice, and The Physiology of Digestion*. Plattsburgh: F. P. Allen.
Beck, C. S. (1935), The development of a new blood supply to the heart by operation. *Ann. Surg.*, 102:801–813.
────── Pritchard, W. H., & Feil, H. S. (1947), Ventricular fibrillation of long duration abolished by electric shock. *J. Amer. Med. Assn.*, 135:985–986.
Beddoes, T., & Watt, J. (1796), *Considerations on the Medicinal Use, and on the Production of Factitious Airs*, Pts. 1, 2. Bristol: J. Johnson.
Berridge, V. (1982), Opiate use in England, 1800–1926. In: *Opioids in Mental Illness: Theories, Clinical Observations, and Treatment Possibilities*, ed. K. Verebey. New York: New York Academy of Sciences, pp. 1–11.
Best, C. H. (1972), Nineteen hundred twenty-one in Toronto. *Diabetes*, 21:385–395.
Beverley, R. (1705), *The History and Present State of Virginia*, Book 2. London: R. Parker.
Beyer, Jr., K. H. (1977), Discovery of the thiazides: Where biology and chemistry meet. *Perspect. Biol. Med.*, 20:410–420.
Biddle, J. B. (1880), *Materia Medica, for the Use of Students*. Philadelphia: Lindsay & Blakiston.
Bigelow, W. G., Lindsay, W. K., & Greenwood, W. F. (1950), Hypothermia—its possible role in cardiac surgery: An investigation of factors governing survival in dogs at low body temperatures. *Ann. Surg.*, 132:849–866.
Bingham, J. B., Meyer, O. O., & Pohle, F. J. (1941), Studies on the hemorrhagic agent 3,3'-methylenebis (4-hydroxycoumarin) 1. Its effect on the prothrombin and coagulation time of the blood of dogs and humans. *Amer. J. Med. Sci.*, 202:563–578.

Black, J. W., Crowther, A. F., Shanks, R. G., Smith, L. H., & Dornhorst, A. C. (1964), A new adrenergic beta-receptor antagonist. *Lancet*, 1:1080–1081.

——— Stephenson, J. S. (1962), Pharmacology of a new adrenergic beta-receptor-blocking compound (nethalide). *Lancet*, 2:311–314.

Black, M. M., Drury, P. J., & Tindale, W. B. (1983), Twenty-five years of heart valve substitutes: A review. *J. Roy. Soc. Med.*, 76:667–680.

Blalock, A., & Taussig, H. B. (1945), The surgical treatment of malformations of the heart in which there is pulmonary stenosis or pulmonary atresia. *J. Amer. Med. Assn.*, 128:189–202.

Bliss, M. (1982), Banting's, Best's, and Collip's accounts of the discovery of insulin. *Bull. Hist. Med.*, 56:554–568.

Blumgart, H. L., Gilligan, D. R., Levy, R. C., Brown, M. G., & Volk, M. C. (1934), Action of diuretic drugs 1. Action of diuretics in normal persons. *Arch. Intern. Med.*, 54:40–81.

Blundell, J. (1818), Experiments on the transfusion of blood by the syringe. *Med.-Chir. Trans.*, 9:56–92.

——— (1828–1829a), Successful case of transfusion. *Lancet*, 1:431–432.

——— (1828–1829b), Observations on transfusion of blood by Dr. Blundell with a description of his Gravitator. *Lancet*, 2:321–324.

Boehm, R. (1878), Ueber Wiederbelebung nach Vergiftungen und Asphyxie. *Arch. Exper. Path. u. Pharmakol.*, 8:68–101.

Booth, J. (1977), A short history of blood pressure measurement. *Proc. Roy. Soc. Med.*, 70:793–799.

Boothby, W. M. (1938), Oxygen administration: The value of high concentration of oxygen for therapy. *Proc. Staff Meetings Mayo Clin.*, 13:641–646.

Borel, J. F., Feurer, C., Gubler, H. U., & Stähelin, H. (1976), Biologic effects of cyclosporin A: A new antilymphocytic agent. *Agents & Actions*, 6:468–475.

Bowditch, H. I. (1846), *The Young Stethoscopist, or the Student's Aid to Auscultation*. Boston: William D. Ticknor & Co.

Boxill, E. H. (1985), *Music Therapy for the Developmentally Disabled*. Rockville, MD: An Aspen Publication.

Bradley, R. (1730), *A Course of Lectures, upon the Materia Medica, Ancient and Modern*. London: Charles Davis.

Braunwald, E. (1966), Symposium on beta adrenergic receptor blockade: An editorial introduction to the symposium. *Amer. J. Cardiol.*, 18:303–307.

Brontë, C. (1846), Evening solace. In: *The Poems of Charlotte Brontë*, ed. T. Winnifrith. Oxford, UK: Basil Blackwell Publisher, Ltd., 1984, pp. 58–59.

Brooks, H. (1928), The use of alcohol in the circulatory defects of old age. *Med. J. Record*, 127:199–201.

Brown, H. M. (1917), The beginnings of intravenous medication. *Ann. Med. Hist.*, 1:177–197.

Bruce, R. A. (1956), Evaluation of functional capacity and exercise tolerance of cardiac patients. *Mod. Concepts Cardiovasc. Dis.*, 25:321–326.

Brunton, T. L. (1867), On the use of nitrite of amyl in angina pectoris. *Lancet*, 2:97–98.

——— (1902), Preliminary note on the possibility of treating mitral stenosis by surgical methods. *Lancet*, 1:352.

——— (1916), On the use of the clinical thermometer. *Lancet*, 1:317.

Bulbulian, A. H. (1938), Design and construction of the masks for the oxygen inhalation apparatus. *Proc. Staff Meetings Mayo Clin.*, 13:654–656.

Bunker, T. D. (1981), The contemporary use of the medicinal leech. *Injury: Brit. J. Accident Surg.*, 12:430–432.

Burch, G. E., & DePasquale, N. P. (1964), *A History of Electrocardiography.* Chicago: Year Book Medical Publishers, Inc.

Burdon-Sanderson, J., & Page, F. J. M. (1880), On the time-relations of the excitatory process in the ventricle of the heart of the frog. *J. Physiol.*, 2:384–435.

Burns, A. (1809), *Observations on Some of the Most Frequent and Important Diseases of the Heart.* Edinburgh: Thomas Bryce & Co.

Cahn, A., & von Mering, J. (1886), Die Sauren des gesunden und kranken Magens. *Deutches Archiv. f. klin. Med.*, 38:233–253.

Callaghan, J. C., & Bigelow, W. G. (1951), An electrical artificial pacemaker for standstill of the heart. *Ann. Surg.*, 134:8–17.

Cammann, G. P. (1855), Editorial: Self-adjusting stethoscope of Dr. Cammann. *New York Med. Times*, 4:140–142.

Campbell, H. A., & Link, K. P. (1941), Studies on the hemorrhagic sweet clover disease IV. The isolation and crystallization of the hemorrhagic agent. *J. Biol. Chem.*, 138:21–33.

Cardinell, R. L. (1948), Music in industry. In: *Music and Medicine*, ed. D. M. Schullian & M. Schoen. New York: Henry Schuman, Inc., pp. 352–366.

Carrel, A., & Guthrie, C. C. (1905), The transplantation of veins and organs. *Amer. Med.*, 10:1101–1102.

Casella, L. P. (1869), Clinical thermometers. *Med. Times & Gazette*, 2:611.

Castle, W. B. (1953), Development of knowledge concerning the gastric intrinsic factor and its relation to pernicious anemia. *New Engl. J. Med.*, 249:603–614.

———— (1961), The Gordon Wilson Lecture: A century of curiosity about pernicious anemia. *Trans. Amer. Clin. Climatol. Assn.*, 73:54–80.

Chapman, C. B. (1967), Edward Smith (?1818–1874): Physiologist, human ecologist, reformer. *J. Hist. Med. Allied Sci.*, 22:1–26.

Chardack, W. M., Gage, A. A., & Greatbatch, W. (1960), A transistorized, self-contained, implantable pacemaker for the long-term correction of complete heart block. *Surgery*, 48:643–654.

Charles, A. F., & Scott, D. A. (1933), Studies on heparin 1. The preparation of heparin. *J. Biol. Chem.*, 102:425–429.

Christian, H. A. (1903), A sketch of the history of the treatment of chlorosis with iron. *Med. Lib. Hist. J.*, 1:176–180.

Cicero (44 B.C.), Cato The Elder on old age (On old age). In: *Cicero—Selected Works*, trans. M. Grant. Middlesex, UK: Penguin Books Ltd., 1971, pp. 211–247.

Clauser, A. R. (1933), The heart tickler or pacemaker. *J. Amer. Med. Assn.*, 100:1628.

Clendening, L. (1935), *Methods of Treatment.* St. Louis: C. V. Mosby Co.

———— (1943), *Behind the Doctor.* New York: Alfred A. Knopf, pp. 20–22.

Combe, J. S. (1824), History of a case of anaemia. *Trans. Med.-Chir. Soc. Edinburgh*, 1:194–204.

Committee on Public Health Relations of the New York Academy of Medicine (1943), Standards of effective administration of inhalation therapy. *J. Amer. Med. Assn.*, 121:755–759.

Comroe, Jr., J. H. (1983), *Exploring the Heart.* New York & London: W. W. Norton & Co.

Congreve, W. (1697), The mourning bride. In: *Masterpieces of the English Drama: William Congreve*, intr. W. Archer. New York, Cincinnati, Chicago: American Book Company, 1912, pp. 367–444.

Conniff, R. (1987), The little suckers have made a comeback. *Discover*, 8:85–94.

Cook, E. N., & Brown, G. E. (1932), The vasodilating effects of ethyl alcohol on the peripheral arteries. *Proc. Staff Meetings Mayo Clin.*, 7:449–452.

Cook, J. D. (1981), The therapeutic use of music: A literature review. *Nursing Forum*, 20:252–266.

Cooper, B. B. (1843), *The Life of Sir Astley Cooper, Bart.*, *Interspersed with Sketches from his Note-books of Distinguished Contemporary Characters*, Vol. 2. London: John W. Parker.

Cooper, D. K. C. (1984), Experimental development and early clinical experience. In: *Heart Transplantation*, ed. D. K. C. Cooper & R. P. Lanza. Lancaster, Boston, The Hague, Dordrecht: MTP Press Limited, pp. 1–14.

——— Lanza, R. P. (1984), Heart transplantations at the University of Capetown—An overview. In: *Heart Transplantation*. ed. D. K. C. Cooper & R. P. Lanza. Lancaster, Boston, The Hague, Dordrecht: MTP Press Limited, pp. 351–360.

Cournand, A. (1964), Air and blood. In: *Circulation of the Blood: Men and Ideas*, ed. A. P. Fishman & D. W. Richards. New York: Oxford University Press, pp. 3–70.

——— Ranges, H. A. (1941), Catheterization of the right auricle in man. *Proc. Soc. Exp. Biol. Med.*, 46:462–466.

Courtwight, D. T. (1982), *Dark Paradise: Opiate Addiction in America before 1940.* Cambridge, MA: Harvard University Press.

Crafoord, C. (1937), Preliminary report on post-operative treatment with heparin as a preventive of thrombosis. *Acta Chir. Scand.*, 79:407–426.

Crile, G. W. (1914), *Anemia and Resuscitation.* New York & London: D. Appleton & Co.

Cummins, B. M., Obetz, S. W., & Wilson, Jr., M. R. (1968), Belladona poisoning as a facet of psychodelia. *J. Amer. Med. Assn.*, 204:1011.

Currie, J. (1804), *Medical Reports, on the Effects of Water, Cold and Warm, as a Remedy in Fever and Other Diseases, Whether applied to the Surface of the Body or used Internally*, Vol. 1. Liverpool: T. Cadell & W. Davies.

Cutler, E. C., & Levine, S. A. (1923), Cardiotomy and valvulotomy for mitral stenonis. Experimental observations and clinical notes concerning an operated case with recovery. *Boston Med. Surg. J.*, 188:1023–1027.

Dale, D. U., & Jaques, L. B. (1942), The prevention of experimental thrombosis by dicoumarin. *Can. Med. Assn. J.*, 46:546–548.

Dale, H. H. (1906), On some physiological actions of ergot. *J. Physiol.*, 34:163–206.

Davison, J. T. R. (1899), Music in medicine. *Lancet*, 2:1159–1162.

DeCastello, A., & Sturli, A. (1902), Ueber die Isoagglutinine im Serum gesunder und kranker Menschen. *München med. Wchnschr.*, 49:1090–1095.

De Quincey, T. (1821), *Confessions of an English Opium-Eater.* Boston: William D. Ticknor, 1841, p. 106.

DeStevens, G. (1963), *Diuretics: Chemistry and Pharmacology.* New York & London: Academic Press.

Dewhurst, J. (1988), Cosmas and Damian, patron saints of doctors. *Lancet*, 2:1479–1480.

Dickey, J. (1970), Diabetes. In: *The Eye-beaters, Blood, Victory, Madness, Buckhead and Mercy.* Garden City, NY: Doubleday & Co., Inc., pp. 7–9.

Dickinson, M. H., & Lent, C. M. (1984), Feeding behavior of the medicinal leech, *Hirudo medicinalis* L. *J. Comp. Physiol. A*, 154:449–455.

Dikshit, R. K. (1980), The story of rauwolfia. *Trends Pharmacol. Sci.*, 1:VIII–X.

Dioscorides, P. (*c.* 77 A.D.), *The Greek Herbal of Dioscorides*, trans. J. Goodyer, ed. R. T. Gunther. London & New York: Hafner Publishing Co., 1968.

Dobson, M. (1776), Experiments and observations on the urine in diabetes. In: *Classic Descriptions of Disease*, ed. R. H. Major. Springfield, IL, & Baltimore, MD: Charles C Thomas, 1932, pp. 195–198.

Dong, Jr., E., Hurley, E. J., Lower, R. R., & Shumway, N. E. (1964), Performance of the heart two years after autotransplantation. *Surgery*, 56:270–274.

Dornhorst, A. C., & Robinson, B. F. (1962), Clinical pharmacology of a beta-adrenergic-blocking agent (nethalide). *Lancet 2*, 2:314–316.

Dover, T. (1733), *The Ancient Physician's Legacy to his Country*. London: A. Betteswoth, C. Hitch & J. Brotherton.

Dryden, J. (1700), To my Honor'd Kinsman, John Driden, of Chesterton, in the County of Huntingdon, Esquire. In: *The Poetical Works of John Dryden*, ed. G. R. Noyes. Boston: Houghton Mifflin Company, 1950, pp. 784–787.

Dussik, K. T., Dussik, F., & Wyt, L. (1947), Auf dem Wege zur Hyperphonographie des Gehirnes. *Wiener Medizinische Wochenschrift*, 97:425–429.

Ebbell, B. (1937), *The Papyrus Ebers: The Greatest Egyptian Medical Document*. Copenhagen: Levin & Munksgaard.

Edelstein, L. (1937), Greek medicine in its relation to religion and magic. *Bull. Inst. Hist. Med.*, 5:201–246.

Edler, I. (1955), The diagnostic use of ultrasound in heart disease. *Acta Med. Scand.* [*Suppl.*], 308:32–36.

———— Hertz, C. H. (1954), The use of ultrasonic reflectoscope for the continuous recording of the movement of heart walls. *Kungl. Fysiografiska Sällskapets i Lund Förhandlingar*, 24, Nr. 5:40–58.

———— ———— (1977), The early work on ultrasound in medicine at the University of Lund. *J. Clin. Ultrasound*, 5:352–356.

Edwards, W. M. (1905), Treatment of disease by music. *Amer. Med.*, 9:305.

Einstein, E. B. (1978), The leech gatherers. *J. Hist. Med. Allied Sci.*, 33:214.

Einthoven, W. (1903), The galvanometric registration of the human electrocardiogram, likewise a review of the use of the capillary-electrometer in physiology. In: *Cardiac Classics*, ed. F. A. Willius & T. E. Keys. St. Louis: C. V. Mosby Co., 1941, pp. 722–728.

———— (1912), The different forms of the human electrocardiogram and their signification. *Lancet*, 1:853–861.

Elders, C. (1925), Tropical sprue and pernicious anaemia: Aetiology and treatment. *Lancet*, 1:75–77.

Ellwanger, G. H. (1897), *Meditations on Gout*. Rutland, VT: George E. Tuttle Co., 1968, p. 23.

Elmqvist, R., Landegren, J., Pettersson, S. D., Senning, A., & William-Olsson, G. (1963), Artificial pacemaker for treatment of Adams-Stokes syndrome and slow heart rate. *Amer. Heart J.*, 65:731–748.

Eloesser, L. (1970), Milestones in chest surgery. *J. Thorac. Cardiovasc. Surg.*, 60:157–165.

Erichsen, J. E. (1881), *The Science and Art of Surgery*, Vol. 1. Philadelphia: Henry C. Lea's Son & Co.

Fahr, G. (1920), An analysis of the spread of the excitation wave in the human ventricle. *Arch. Intern. Med.*, 25:146–173.

Fairbanks, V. F., Fahey, J. L., & Beutler, E. (1971), *Clinical Disorders of Iron Metabolism*. New York & London: Grune & Stratton.

Faivre, J. (1856), Pathological physiology: Experimental studies on the organic lesions of the heart. In: *Classics in Arterial Hypertension*, ed. A. Ruskin. Springfield, IL: Charles C Thomas, 1956, pp. 67–73.

Fantus, B. (1937), The therapy of the Cook County Hospital: Blood preservation. *J. Amer. Med. Assn.*, 109:128–131.

Feigenbaum, H. (1972), *Echocardiography*. Philadelphia: Lea & Febiger.

Feil, H., & Siegel, M. L. (1928), Electrocardiographic changes during attacks of angina pectoris. *Amer. J. Med. Sci.*, 175:255–260.

Fenwick, S. (1870), On atrophy of the stomach. *Lancet*, 2:78–80.

Field, A. G. (1858), On the toxical and medicinal properties of nitrate of oxyde of glycyl. *Med. Times & Gazette*, 16:291–292.

Firestone, F. A. (1946), The supersonic reflectoscope, an instrument for inspecting the interior of solid parts by means of sound waves. *J. Acoust. Soc. Amer.*, 17:287–299.

Flint, A. (1862), On cardiac murmurs. *Amer. J. Med. Sci.*, 44:29–54.

——— (1866), Remarks on the use of the thermometer in diagnosis and prognosis. *New York Med. J.*, 4:81–93.

Forbes, T. R. (1977), Why is it called "beautiful lady"? A note on belladona. *Bull. New York Acad. Med.*, 53:403–406.

Forssmann, W. (1929), Die Sondierung des rechten Herzens [Catheterization of the right heart]. In: *Classics of Cardiology*, Vol. 3. ed. J. A. Callahan, T. E. Keys, & J. D. Key. Malabar, FL: Robert E. Krieger Publishing Co., 1983, pp. 252–255.

Fothergill, J. (1745), Observations on a case published in the last volume of the medical essays, etc. of recovering a man dead in appearance, by distending the lungs with air. *Philos. Trans. Roy. Soc. Lond.*, 43:275–281.

Fowler, W. M. (1936), Chlorosis—An obituary. *Ann. Med. Hist.*, N.S. 8:168–177.

Fox III, S. M., & Skinner, J. S. (1964), Physical activity and cardiovascular health. *Amer. J. Cardiol.*, 14:731–746.

Furman, S., & Robinson, G. (1958), The use of an intracardiac pacemaker in the correction of total heart block. *Surg. Forum*, 9:245–248.

——— Schwedel, J. B. (1959), An intracardiac pacemaker for Stokes-Adams seizures. *New Engl. J. Med.*, 261:943–948.

Galvani, L. (1791), *Commentary on the Effects of Electricity on Muscular Motion*, intr. I. B. Cohen, trans. M. G. Foley [Ames]. Norwalk, CT: Burndy Library, 1953.

Ganorkar, S. W., & Mandal, H. V. P. (1973), Medicine and physical exercise in ancient India. *J. Sports Med. Phys. Fitness*, 13:134–136.

Garrison, F. H. (1929), *An Introduction to the History of Medicine*. Philadelphia & London: W. B. Saunders Co.

Garrod, A. B. (1876), *A Treatise on Gout and Rheumatic Gout*. London: Longmans, Green, & Co.

Gerarde, J. (1597), *The Herball or General Historie of Plantes*. London: John Norton.

Gibbon, Jr., J. H. (1954), Application of a mechanical heart and lung apparatus to cardiac surgery. *Minnesota Med.*, 37:171–180, 185.

Goldsmith, S. R., Frank, I., & Ungerleider, J. T. (1968), Poisoning from ingestion of a stramonium-belladona mixture. *J. Amer. Med. Assn.*, 204:169–170.

Graham, E. A. (1957), A brief account of the development of thoracic surgery and some of its consequences. *Surg. Gynecol. Obstet.*, 104:241–250.

Gray, H. M. W. (1905), Subdiaphragmatic transperitoneal massage of the heart as a means of resuscitation. *Lancet*, 2:506.

Green, C., & Gilby, J. A. (1983), The medicinal leech. *J. Roy. Soc. Health*, 103:42–44.

Green, T. A. (1906), Heart massage as a means of restoration in cases of apparent sudden death, with a synopsis of 40 cases. *Lancet*, 2:1708–1714.

Greenberg, L. A., & Carpenter, J. A. (1957), The effect of alcoholic beverages on skin conductance and emotional tension 1. Wine, whiskey and alcohol. *Quart. J. Stud. Alc.*, 18:190–204.

Gross, R. E., & Hubbard, J. P. (1939), Surgical ligation of a patent ductus arteriosus: Report of first successful case. *J. Amer. Med. Assn.*, 112:729–731.

Gurvich, N. L., & Yuniev, G. S. (1946), Restoration of regular rhythm in the mammalian fibrillating heart. *Amer. Rev. Soviet Med.*, 3:236–239.

——— ——— (1947), Restoration of heart rhythm during fibrillation by a condenser discharge. *Amer. Rev. Soviet Med.*, 4:252–256.

Habershon, S. O. (1866), Clinical remarks on the treatment of diseases of the heart. *Guy's Hosp. Reports*, 12 (3rd Series): 303–327.

Haden, R. L. (1938), Historical aspects of iron therapy in anemia. *J. Amer. Med. Assn.*, 111:1059–1061.

Haggis, A. W. (1941), Fundamental errors in the early history of cinchona. *Bull. Hist. Med.*, 10:568–592.

Hake, T. G. (1874), Studies on ether and chloroform, from Prof. Schiff's physiological laboratory. *The Practitioner*, 12:241–250.

Haldane, J. S. (1917), The therapeutic administration of oxygen. *Brit. Med. J.*, 1:181–183.

——— Kellas, A. M., & Kennaway, E. L. (1919), Experiments on acclimatisation to reduced atmospheric pressure. *J. Physiol.*, 53:181–206.

Hales, S. (1733), *Statical Essays: Containing Haemastatics*, Vol. 2. London: Wilson & Nicol, 1769.

Haller, Jr., J. S. (1981), Hypodermic medication: Early history. *New York State J. Med.*, 81:1671–1679.

——— (1985), Medical thermometry—A short history. *West. J. Med.*, 142:108–116.

Hamilton, W. F., & Richards, D. W. (1964), The output of the heart. In: *Circulation of the Blood: Men and Ideas*, ed. A. P. Fishman & D. W. Richards. New York: Oxford University Press, pp. 71–126.

Hanzlik, P. J. (1929), 125th anniversary of the discovery of morphine by Sertürner. *J. Amer. Pharm. Assn.*, 18:375–384.

Hardy, J. D., Chavez, C. M., Kurrus, F. D., Neely, W. A., Eraslan, S., Turner, M. D., Fabian, L. W., & Labecki, T. D. (1964), Heart transplantation in man: Developmental studies and report of a case. *J. Amer. Med. Assn.*, 188:1132–1140.

Hare, F. E. (1891), Quinine as a cardiac stimulant. *Lancet*, 1:930–931.

Harford, F. K. (1891), Music in illness. *Lancet*, 2:43–44.

Harken, D. E., & Curtis, L. E. (1967), Heart surgery—Legend and a long look. *Amer. J. Cardiol.*, 19:393–400.

——— Ellis, L. B., Ware, P. F., & Norman, L. R. (1948), The surgical treatment of mitral stenosis I. Valvuloplasty. *New Engl. J. Med.*, 239:801–809.

——— Soroff, H. S., Taylor, W. J., Lefemine, A. A., Gupta, S. K., & Lunzer, S. (1960), Partial and complete prostheses in aortic insufficiency. *J. Thorac. Cardiovasc. Surg.*, 40:744–762.

Hartung, E. F. (1954), History of the use of colchicum and related medicaments in gout. *Ann. Rheum. Dis.*, 13:190–200.

Hay, J. (1924), The action of quinidine in the treatment of heart disease. *Lancet*, 2:543–545.

Haycraft, J. B. (1884), On the action of a secretion obtained from the medicinal leech on the coagulation of the blood. *Proc. Roy. Soc. London*, 36:478–487.

Hayter, A. (1968), *Opium and the Romantic Imagination*. Berkeley & Los Angeles: University of California Press.

Heath, C. W., Strauss, M. B., & Castle, W. B. (1932), Quantitative aspects of iron deficiency in hypochromic anemia. *J. Clin. Invest.*, 11:1293–1312.

Heberden, W. (1802), *Commentaries on the History and Cure of Diseases*. London: T. Payne.

Heiser, Jr., C. B. (1969), *Nightshades: The Paradoxical Plants*. San Francisco: W. H. Freeman & Co.

Henderson, L. J. (1928), *Blood: A Study in General Physiology*. New Haven: Yale University Press.

Herrick, J. B. (1919), Thrombosis of the coronary arteries. *J. Amer. Med. Assn.*, 72:387–390.

Hertz, C. H. (1973), The interaction of physicians, physicists and industry in the development of echocardiography. *Ultrasound Med. Biol.*, 1:3–11.

Hicks, J. B. (1869), Cases of transfusion, with some remarks on a new method of performing the operation. *Guy's Hosp. Reports*, 14 (3rd Series):1–14.

Hicky, D. W. (n.d.), No friend like music. In: *Poems That Touch The Heart*, comp. A. L. Alexander. Garden City, NY: Doubleday & Company, Inc., 1956.

Hill, L. (1921), A simple oxygen bed tent and its use to a case of oedema and chronic ulcer of the leg. In: Proceedings of the Physiological Society, March 21, 1921, *J. Physiol.*, 55:xx–xxi.

—— Barnard, H. (1897), A simple and accurate form of sphygmometer or arterial pressure gauge contrived for clinical use. *Brit. Med. J.*, 2:904.

Hippocrates (c. 400 B.C.a), *The Genuine Works of Hippocrates*, Vol. 1, trans. F. Adams. London: The Sydenham Society, 1849.

—— (c. 400 B.C.b), *The Genuine Works of Hippocrates*, Vol. 2, trans. F. Adams. London: The Sydenham Society, 1849.

Hodgkin, D. C., Kamper, J., Mackay, M., Pickworth, J., Trueblood, K. N., & White, J. G. (1956), Structure of vitamin B_{12}. *Nature*, 178:64–66.

Holmes, J. H. (1980), Diagnostic ultrasound during the early years of A.I.U.M. *J. Clin. Ultrasound.*, 8:299–308.

Holmes, O. W. (1849), The Stethoscope Song. In: *Poems by Oliver Wendell Holmes*. Boston: William D. Ticknor & Co., pp. 258–263.

Holmes, R. W., & Love, J. (1952), Suicide attempt with warfarin, a bishydroxycoumarin-like rodenticide. *J. Amer. Med. Assn.*, 148:935–937.

Hooke, R. (1705), *The Posthumous Works of Robert Hooke*, intr. R. S. Westfall. New York & London: Johnson Reprint Corporation, 1969.

Hooker, D. R., Kouwenhoven, W. B., & Langworthy, O. R. (1933), The effect of alternating electrical currents on the heart. *Amer. J. Physiol.*, 103:444–454.

Hope, J. (1832), *A Treatise on the Diseases of the Heart and Great Vessels*. London: W. Kidd.

Howard-Jones, N. (1947), A critical study of the origins and early development of hypodermic medication. *J. Hist. Med.*, 2:201–249.

Howell, M., & Ford, P. (1985), *Medical Mysteries*. Harmondsworth, Middlesex, UK: Viking, Penguin Books Ltd., pp. 210–236.

Howell, W. H., & Holt, E. (1918), Two new factors in blood coagulation—heparin and pro-antithrombin. *Amer. J. Physiol.*, 47:328–341.

Hufnagel, C. A. (1951), Aortic plastic valvular prosthesis. *Bull. Georgetown Univ. Med. Center*, 4:128–130.

—— (1979), Basic concepts in the development of cardiovascular prostheses. *Amer. J. Surg.*, 137:285–300.

—— Harvey, W. P. (1953), The surgical correction of aortic regurgitation: Preliminary report. *Bull. Georgetown Univ. Med. Center*, 6:60–61.

—— —— Rabil, P. J., & McDermott, T. F. (1954), Surgical correction of aortic insufficiency. *Surgery*, 35:673–683.

Hunter, C. (1859), A series of cases of narcotic injection into the cellular tissue in neuralgia and other diseases. *Brit. Med. J.*, 1859:19–20.

Hunter, J. E. (1892), Is soft music a calmative in cases of fever? *Lancet*, 2:923.

Huser, H.-J. (1966), A note on Biermer's anemia. *Med. Clin. North Amer.*, 50:1611–1626.

Husson, N. (1783), *Collection de Faits et Recueil d'Expériences sur le Spécifique et les Effets de l'Eau Médicinale*. Bouillon: J. Brasseur.

Hustin, A. (1914), Principe d'une nouvelle méthod de transfusion muqueuse. *J. Méd. Brux.*, 12:436–439.

Hutchin, P. (1968), History of blood transfusion: A tercentennial look. *Surgery*, 64:685–700.

Hyde, I. H. (1924), Effects of music upon electrocardiograms and blood pressure. *J. Exp. Psychol.*, 7:213–224.

Hyde, R. W., & Rawson, A. J. (1969), Unintentional iatrogenic oxygen pneumonitis—Response to therapy. *Ann. Intern. Med.*, 71:517–531.

Hyman, A. S. (1932), Resuscitation of the stopped heart by intracardial therapy. II. Experimental use of an artificial pacemaker. *Arch. Intern. Med.*, 50:283–305.

Jackson, J. (1827), *Textbook of a Course of Lectures, on the Theory and Practice of Physic. Part Second. For the Use of the Medical Students of Harvard University.* Boston: Wells & Lilly.

James, W. B., & Williams, H. B. (1910), The electrocardiogram in clinical medicine. *Amer. J. Med. Sci.*, 140:408–421.

Johnson, J. R. (1816), *A Treatise on The Medicinal Leech; Including its Medical and Natural History, with a Description of its Anatomical Structure; also, Remarks upon the Diseases, Preservation and Management of Leeches.* London: Longman, Hurst, Rees, Orme & Brown.

Johnson, S. L. (1970), *The History of Cardiac Surgery, 1896–1955.* Baltimore and London: The Johns Hopkins Press.

Jones, P. M. (1984), *Medieval Medical Miniatures*. London: British Library Reference Division Publications.

Jonkman, E. J. (1980), An historical note: Doppler research in the nineteenth century. *Ultrasound Med. Biol.*, 6:1–5.

Katz, L. N., & Hellerstein, H. K. (1964), Electrocardiography. In: *Circulation of the Blood: Men and Ideas*, ed. A. P. Fishman & D. W. Richards. New York: Oxford University Press, pp. 265–351.

Kay, C. F. (1966), Quinidine—A re-evaluation. *Med. Clin. North Amer.*, 50:1221–1230.

Keats, J. (1819), To Sleep. In: *The Complete Poetical Works of Keats*, ed. H. E. Scudder. Boston: Houghton Mifflin Company, 1899, p. 142.

Kilmer, F. B. (1925), Rambling among the nightshades. *Amer. J. Pharm.*, 97:4–38.

Klein, M. D., Barret, J., Ryan, T. J., & Flessas, A. P. (1975), Atropine dose in acute myocardial infarction in man. *Cardiology*, 60:193–205.

Koff, M. (1966), Poisoning from ingestion of asthma "powders." *J. Amer. Med. Assn.*, 198:1034.

Kondo, Y., Grädel, F., & Kantrowitz, A. (1965), Heart homotransplantation in puppies: Long survival without immunosuppressive therapy. *Circulation*, 31 (Suppl. 1):1-181–1-187.

Korotkov, N. S. (1905), A contribution to the problem of methods for the determination of the blood pressure. In: *Classics in Arterial Hyptertension*, ed. A. Ruskin, Springfield, IL: Charles C Thomas, 1956, pp. 127–133.

Kouwenhoven, W. B. (1969), The development of the defibrillator. *Ann. Intern. Med.*, 71:449–458.

———— Jude, J. R., & Knickerbocker, G. G. (1960), Closed-chest cardiac massage. *J. Amer. Med. Assn.*, 173:1064–1067.

———— Langworthy, O. R. (1973), Cardiopulmonary resuscitation: An account of forty-five years of research. *Johns Hopkins Med. J.*, 132:186–193.

———— Milnor, W. R., Knickerbocker, G. G., & Chesnut, W. R. (1957), Closed chest defibrillation of the heart. *Surgery*, 42:550–561.

Kramer, J. C. (1980), The opiates: Two centuries of scientific study. *J. Psychedelic Drugs*, 12:89–103.

Kramer, S. N. (1954), First pharmacopeia in man's recorded history. *Amer. J. Pharm.*, 126:76–84.

Krantz, Jr., J. C. (1975), Historical background. In: *Organic Nitrates*, ed. P. Needleman. New York, Heidelberg, Berlin: Springer-Verlag, 1975, pp. 1–13.

Krause, A. C. (1934), Assyro-Babylonian ophthalmology. *Ann. Med. Hist.*, N.S. 6:42–55.

Kreig, M. B. (1964), *Green Medicine: The Search For Plants That Heal.* . . . Chicago, New York, San Francisco: Rand McNally & Co.

Laënnec, R. T. H. (1819), *Traité de l'auscultation médiate* [A Treatise on the Diseases of the Chest], trans. J. Forbes. Philadelphia: J. Webster, 1823.

Lands, A. M., Arnold, A., McAuliff, J. P., Luduena, F. P., & Brown, Jr., T. G. (1967), Differentiation of receptor systems activated by sympathomimetic amines. *Nature*, 214:597–598.

Landsteiner, K. (1901), Ueber Agglutinations-erscheinungen normalen menschlichen Blutes. *Wien. klin. Wchnschr.*, 14:1132–1134.

———— (1931), Individual differences in human blood. *Science*, 73:403–409.

Lange, J. (1554), Medicinalium epistolarum miscellanea. In: *Classic Descriptions of Disease*, ed. R. H. Major. Springfield, IL, & Baltimore, MD: Charles C Thomas, 1932, pp. 445–447.

Langley, J. N. (1906), Croonian Lecture, 1906.—On nerve endings and on special excitable substances in cells. *Proc. Roy. Soc. Lond.*, 78B:170–194.

Latham, P. M. (1861), General remarks on the practice of medicine IV. Cure. *Brit. Med. J.*, 2:323–325.

Lawrence, C. (1979), Physiological apparatus in the Wellcome Museum. 3. Early sphygmomanometers. *Med. Hist.*, 23:474–478.

Leake, C. D. (1952), *The Old Egyptian Medical Papyri*. Lawrence, Kansas: University of Kansas Press.

Lent, C. M. (1985), Serotonergic modulation of the feeding behavior of the medicinal leech. *Brain Res. Bull.*, 14:643–655.

————— (1986), New medicinal and scientific uses of the leech. *Nature*, 323:494.

Levine, S. A., & Harvey, W. P. (1959), *Clinical Auscultation of the Heart*. Philadelphia & London: W. B. Saunders Co.

Levinthal, C. F. (1985), Milk of paradise/milk of hell—the history of ideas about opium. *Perspect. Biol. Med.*, 28:561–577.

Lewis, T. (1912), Electro-cardiography and its importance in the clinical examination of heart affections. *Brit. Med. J.*, 2:65–67.

————— (1915), *Lectures on the Heart*. New York: Paul B. Hoeber.

————— Drury, A. N., Iliescu, C. C., & Wedd, A. M. (1921), The manner in which quinidine sulphate acts in auricular fibrillation. *Brit. Med. J.*, 2:514–515.

Lewis, Jr., W. H. (1941), The evolution of clinical sphygmomanometry. *Bull. New York Acad. Med.*, 17:871–881.

Lewisohn, R. (1916), The importance of the proper dosage of sodium citrate in blood transfusion. *Ann. Surg.*, 64:618–623.

Licht, S. (1965), History. In: *Therapeutic Exercise*, ed. S. Licht. New Haven, CT: Elizabeth Licht, Publisher, pp. 426–471.

Link, K. P. (1959), The discovery of dicumarol and its sequels. *Circulation*, 19:97–107.

Litwak, R. S. (1971), The growth of cardiac surgery: Historical notes. *Cardiovasc. Clin.*, 3, No. 2:5–50.

Lockemann, G. (1951), Friedrich Wilhelm Sertürner, the discoverer of morphine. *J. Chem. Educ.*, 28:277–279.

Lovelace, II, W. R. (1938), Oxygen for therapy and aviation: An apparatus for the administration of oxygen or oxygen and helium by inhalation. *Proc. Staff Meetings Mayo Clin.*, 13:646–654.

Lower, R. (1669), Tractatus de Corde, trans. K. J. Franklin. In: R. T. Gunther, *Early Science in Oxford*, Vol. IX. Oxford: Printed for the Subscribers, 1932.

Lower, R. R., Dong, Jr., E., & Shumway, N. E. (1965), Long-term survival of cardiac homografts. *Surgery*, 58:110–119.

————— Shumway, N. E. (1960), Studies on orthotopic homotransplantation of the canine heart. *Surg. Forum*, 11:18–19.

Lucia, S. P. (1963a), *A History of Wine as Therapy*. Philadelphia & Montreal: J. B. Lippincott Co.

————— (1963b), Balm for the autumnal years. *Western Med.*, 4:170–171, 178.

Ludwig, C. (1847), Contributions to the knowledge of the influence of the respiratory movements upon the blood flow in the arterial system. In: *Classics in Arterial Hypertension*, ed. A. Ruskin. Springfield, IL: Charles C Thomas, 1956, pp. 61–66.

Macdonald, J. (1909), An address on the remediable use of alcohol. *Brit. Med. J.*, 1:265–268.

Mackenzie, J. (1910), *Diseases of the Heart*. New York: Oxford University Press, pp. 67–74.

Macleod, J. J. R. (1978), History of the researches leading to the discovery of insulin. *Bull. Hist. Med.*, 52:295–312.

Maitland, D. (1982), *5000 Years of Tea*. New York: Gallery Books, imprint of W. H. Smith Publishers Inc.

Major, R. H. (1930), The history of taking the blood pressure. *Ann. Med. Hist.*, N.S. 2:47–55.

————— (1954a), *A History of Medicine*, Vol. 1. Springfield, IL: Charles C Thomas.

————— (1954b), *A History of Medicine*, Vol. 2. Springfield, IL: Charles C Thomas.

Maluf, N. S. R. (1954), History of blood transfusion. *J. Hist. Med.*, 9:59–107.

Mann, F. C., Priestley, J. T., Markowitz, J., & Yater, W. M. (1933), Transplantation of the intact mammalian heart. *Arch. Surg.*, 26:219–224.

Marcus, E., Wong, S. N. T., & Luisada, A. A. (1951), Homologous heart grafts: Transplantation of the heart in dogs. *Surg. Forum*, 2:212–217.

Martindale, W. H., & Westcott, W. W. (1904), *The Extra Pharmacopoeia of Martindale and Westcott.* London: H. K. Lewis.

Mason, C. (1978), Musical activities with elderly patients. *Physiotherapy*, 64:80–82.

Massey, R. U. (1987), Reflections on medicine: History, hot and cold. *Conn. Med.*, 51:755.

Master, A. M., & Oppenheimer, E. T. (1929), A simple exercise tolerance test for circulatory efficiency with standard tables for normal individuals. *Amer. J. Med. Sci.*, 177:223–242.

Maugham, W. S. (1915), *Of Human Bondage.* Garden City, NY: Doubleday & Company, Inc., 1936.

McGuigan, H. (1921), The effect of small doses of atropin on the heart rate. *J. Amer. Med. Assn.*, 76:1338–1340.

McLean, J. (1916), The thromboplastic action of cephalin. *Amer. J. Physiol.*, 41:250–257.

——— (1959), The discovery of heparin. *Circulation*, 19:75–78.

McWilliam, J. A. (1887), Fibrillar contraction of the heart. *J. Physiol.*, 8:296–310.

——— (1889), Electrical stimulation of the heart in man. *Brit. Med. J.*, 1:348–350.

——— Melvin, G. S. (1914), Systolic and diastolic blood pressure estimation, with special reference to the auditory method. *Brit. Med. J.*, 1:693–697.

Meakins, J. (1921), Observations on the gases in human arterial blood in certain pathological pulmonary conditions, and their treatment with oxygen. *J. Pathol. Bacteriol.*, 24:79–90.

Meinecke, B. (1948), Music and medicine in classical antiquity. In: *Music and Medicine*, ed. D. M. Schullian & M. Schoen. New York: Henry Schuman, Inc., pp. 47–95.

Meltzer, S. J. (1917), The therapeutic value of oral rhythmic insufflation of oxygen. *J. Amer. Med. Assn.*, 69:1150–1156.

——— Auer, J. (1909), Continuous respiration without respiratory movements. *J. Exp. Med.*, 11:622–625.

Mettler, C. C. (1947), *History of Medicine*, ed. F. A. Mettler. Philadelphia & Toronto: The Blakiston Co.

Meulengracht, E. (1923), Large doses of iron in the different kinds of anaemia in a medical department. *Acta. Med. Scand.*, 58:594–611.

Miller, A. H. (1931), The Pneumatic Institution of Thomas Beddoes at Clifton, 1798. *Ann. Med. Hist.*, N.S. 3:253–260.

Minot, G. R., & Murphy, W. P. (1926), Treatment of pernicious anemia by a special diet. *J. Amer. Med. Assn.*, 87:470–476.

Monachino, J. (1954), Rauvolfia serpentina—Its history, botany and medical use. *Econ. Bot.*, 8:349–365.

Moran, N. C., & Perkins, M. E. (1958), Adrenergic blockade of the mammalian heart by a dichloro analogue of isoproterenol. *J. Pharmacol. Exp. Ther.*, 124:223–237.

——— ——— (1961), An evaluation of adrenergic blockade of the mammalian heart. *J. Pharmacol. Exp. Ther.*, 133:192–201.

Morris, J. N., & Crawford, M. D. (1958), Coronary heart disease and physical activity of work. *Brit. Med. J.*, 2:1485–1496.

Morton, H. J. V., & Thomas, E. T. (1958), Effect of atropine on the heart-rate. *Lancet*, 2:1313–1315.

Munch, J. C., & Petter, H. H. (1965), The story of glyceryl trinitrate . . . development of glonoin. *J. Amer. Pharm. Assn.*, N. S. 5:491, 494.

Munro, J. C. (1907), Surgery of the vascular system 1. Ligation of the ductus arteriosus. *Ann. Surg.*, 46:335–338.

Munro, S., & Mount, B. (1978), Music therapy in palliative care. *Can. Med. Assn. J.*, 119:1029–1034.

Murray, D. W. G., Jaques, L. B., Perrett, T. S., & Best, C. H. (1937), Heparin and the thrombosis of veins following injury. *Surgery*, 2:163–187.

Murray, I. (1969), The search for insulin. *Scott. Med. J.*, 14:286–293.

———— (1971), Paulesco and the isolation of insulin. *J. Hist. Med. Allied Sci.*, 26:150–157.

Murrell, W. (1879a), Nitro-glycerine as a remedy for angina pectoris. *Lancet*, 1:80–81.

———— (1879b), Nitro-glycerine as a remedy for angina pectoris. *Lancet*, 1:113–115.

———— (1879c), Nitro-glycerine as a remedy for angina pectoris. *Lancet*, 1:151–152.

———— (1879d), Nitro-glycerine as a remedy for angina pectoris. *Lancet*, 1:225–227.

Nickerson, M., & Goodman, L. S. (1947), Pharmacological properties of a new adrenergic blocking agent: N,N-dibenzyl-β-chloroethylamine (Dibenamine). *J. Pharmacol. Exp. Ther.*, 89:167–185.

Novello, F. C., & Sprague, J. M. (1957), Benzothiadiazine dioxides as novel diuretics. *J. Amer. Chem. Soc.*, 79:2028–2029.

Opie, E. L. (1901), Diabetes mellitus associated with hyaline degeneration of the islets of Langerhans of the pancreas. *Johns Hopkins Hosp. Bull.*, 12:263–264.

O'Shaughnessy, L. (1937), Surgical treatment of cardiac ischaemia. *Lancet*, 1:185–194.

Osler, W. (1896), Thomas Dover, M. B. (of Dover's Powder), physician and buccaneer. *Johns Hopkins Hosp. Bull.*, 7:1–6.

Osol, A., & Farrar, Jr., G. E. (1947), *The Dispensatory of the United States of America—The 24th Edition*. Philadelphia: J. B. Lippincott Company.

Ottenberg, R. (1908), Transfusion and arterial anastomosis. *Ann. Surg.*, 47:486–505.

———— Kaliski, D. J. (1913), Accidents in transfusion. *J. Amer. Med. Assn.*, 61:2138–2140.

Palarea, E. R. (1963), Some physiologic effects of ethyl alcohol and their application in modern therapeutics. *J. Amer. Geriat. Soc.*, 11:933–944.

Pantridge, J. F., & Geddes, J. S. (1967), A mobile intensive-care unit in the management of myocardial infarction. *Lancet*, 2:271–273.

Pardee, H. E. B. (1920), An electrocardiographic sign of coronary artery obstruction. *Arch. Intern. Med.*, 26:244–257.

Parsonnet, V., Zucker, I. R., & Asa, M. (1962), Preliminary investigation of the development of a permanent implantable pacemaker utilizing an intracardiac dipolar electrode. *Clin. Res.*, 10:391.

Patz, A., Hoeck, L. E., & De La Cruz, E. (1952), Studies on the effect of high oxygen administration in retrolental fibroplasia. *Amer. J. Ophthalmol.*, 35:1248–1253.

Paulshock, B. Z. (1983), William Heberden and opium—Some relief to all. *New Engl. J. Med.*, 308:53–56.

Payton, B. (1981a), History of medicinal leeching and early medical references. In:

Neurobiology of the Leech, ed. K. J. Muller, J. G. Nicholls, & G. S. Stent. New York: Cold Spring Harbor Laboratory, pp. 27–34.

———— (1981b), Structure of the leech nervous system. In: *Neurobiology of the Leech*, ed. K. J. Muller, J. G. Nicholls, & G. S. Stent. New York: Cold Spring Harbor Laboratory, pp. 35–50.

———— (1984), An historical survey of illustrations of the medicinal leech. *J. Audiov. Media Med.*, 7:105–112.

Pennock, J. L., Oyer, P. E., Reitz, B. A., Jamieson, S. W., Bieber, C. P., Wallwork, J., Stinson, E. B., & Shumway, N. E. (1982), Cardiac transplantation in perspective for the future: Survival, complications, rehabilitation, and cost. *J. Thorac. Cardiovasc. Surg.*, 83:168–177.

Pepys, S. (1666–1668), *Diary and Correspondence of Samuel Pepys, F.R.S.*, Vol. 3, ed. R. L. Braybrooke. London: Henry G. Bohn, 1858.

Pfeiffer, C. J. (1985), *The Art and Practice of Western Medicine in the Early Nineteenth Century*. Jefferson, NC, & London: McFarland & Company, Inc., Publishers.

Pinel, P. (1806), *A Treatise on Insanity*, trans. D. D. Davis. Sheffield: Cadell & Davies.

Plath, S. (1961), The Surgeon at 2 a.m. In: *The Collected Poems: Sylvia Plath*, ed. T. Hughes. New York: Harper & Row, 1981, pp. 170–171.

Plautus, T. M. (c. 200 B.C.), The Comedy of Asses. In: *The Complete Roman Drama*, Vol. 1, ed. G. E. Duckworth. New York: Random House, 1942, pp. 59–111.

Pope, A. (n.d.), Epistle to Dr. Arbuthnot. In: *The Complete Poetical Works of Pope*, ed. H. W. Boynton. Boston: Houghton Mifflin Company, 1931, pp. 176–182.

Powell, C. E., & Slater, I. H. (1958), Blocking of inhibitory adrenergic receptors by a dichloro analog of isoproterenol. *J. Pharmacol. Exp. Ther.*, 122:480–488.

Quick, A. J. (1937), The coagulation defect in sweet clover disease and in the hemorrhagic chick disease of dietary origin. *Amer. J. Physiol.*, 118:260–271.

———— Stanley-Brown, M., & Bancroft, F. W. (1935), A study of the coagulation defect in hemophilia and in jaundice. *Amer. J. Med. Sci.*, 190:501–511.

Rao, P., Bailie, F. B., & Bailey, B. N. (1985), Leechmania in microsurgery. *The Practitioner*, 229:901–905.

Rehn, L. (1897), Ueber penetrirende Herzwunden und Herznaht [Penetrating cardiac wounds and cardiac suture]. In: *Classics of Cardiology*, Vol. 3, ed. J. A. Callahan, T. E. Keys, & J. D. Key. Malabar, FL: Robert E. Krieger Publishing Co., 1983, pp. 36–44.

Richards, Jr., D. W. (1962), Medical priesthoods, past and present. *Trans. Assn. Amer. Physicians*, 75:1–10.

———— Cournand, A., Darling, R. C., Gillespie, W. H., & Baldwin, E. DeF. (1942), Pressure of blood in the right auricle, in animals and in man: Under normal conditions and in right heart failure. *Amer. J. Physiol.*, 136:115–123.

Rickes, E. L., Brink, N. G., Koniuszy, F. R., Wood, T. R., & Folkers, K. (1948), Crystalline vitamin B_{12}. *Science*, 107:396–397.

Robertson, O. H. (1918), Transfusion with preserved red blood cells. *Brit. Med. J.*, 1:691–695.

Roderick, L. M. (1931), A problem in the coagulation of the blood: "Sweet clover disease of cattle." *Amer. J. Physiol.*, 96:413–425.

Rodnan, G. P., & Benedek, T. G. (1963), Ancient therapeutic arts in the gout. *Arthritis Rheum.*, 6:317–340.

—— —— (1970), The early history of antirheumatic drugs. *Arthritis Rheum.*, 13:145–165.

Rolleston, H. D. (1909), Discussion on the treatment of oedema. *Brit. Med. J.*, 2:536–539.

—— (1924), Alcohol in medicine. *The Practitioner*, 113:209–215.

Rous, P., & Turner, J. R. (1916), The preservation of living red blood cells in vitro 1. Methods of preservation. *J. Exp. Med.*, 23:219–237.

Rynd, F. (1845), Neuralgia—Introduction of fluid to the nerve. *Dublin Med. Press*, 13:167–168.

—— (1861), Description of an instrument for the subcutaneous introduction of fluids in affections of the nerves. *Dublin Quarterly J. Med. Sci.*, 32:13.

Safar, P., Escarraga, L. A., & Elam, J. O., (1958), A comparison of the mouth-to-mouth and mouth-to-airway methods of artificial respiration with the chest-pressure arm-lift methods. *New Engl. J. Med.*, 258:671–677.

Samways, D. W. (1898), Cardiac peristalsis: Its nature and effects. *Lancet*, 1:927.

Sanger, F. (1960), Chemistry of insulin. *Brit. Med. Bull.*, 16:183–188.

Satomura, S. (1957), Ultrasonic Doppler method for the inspection of cardiac functions. *J. Acoust. Soc. Amer.*, 29:1181–1185.

Saunders, J. B. deC. M. (1972), A conceptual history of transplantation. In: *Transplantation*, ed. J. S. Najarian & R. L. Simmons. Philadelphia: Lea & Febiger, pp. 3–25.

Schäfer, E. A. (1895), Address in physiology: On internal secretion. *Brit. Med. J.*, 2:341–348.

—— (1908), Artificial respiration in man. In: *Harvey Lectures 1907–1908*. Philadelphia & London: J. B. Lippincott, 1909, pp. 223–243.

Schechter, D. C. (1971a), Early experience with resuscitation by means of electricity. *Surgery*, 69:360–372.

—— (1971b), Background of clinical cardiac electrostimulation. I. Responsiveness of quiescent, bare heart to electricity. *New York State J. Med.*, 71:2575–2581.

—— (1972a), Background of clinical cardiac electrostimulation. IV. Early studies on feasibility of accelerating heart rate by means of electricity. *New York State J. Med.*, 72:395–404.

—— (1972b), Background of clinical cardiac electrostimulation. V. Direct electrostimulation of heart without thoracotomy. *New York State J. Med.*, 72:605–619.

Schnitker, M. A. (1936), A history of the treatment of gout. *Bull. Hist. Med.*, 4:89–120.

Schofield, F. W. (1924), Damaged sweet clover: The cause of a new disease in cattle simulating hemorrhagic septicemia and blackleg. *J. Amer. Vet. Med. Assn.*, 64:553–575.

Schultes, R. E., & Hofmann, A. (1979), *Plants of the Gods*. New York, St. Louis, San Francisco: McGraw-Hill Book Co.

—— —— (1980), *The Botany and Chemistry of Hallucinogens*. Springfield, IL: Charles C Thomas.

Schwartz, R., Stack, J., & Damashek, W. (1958), Effect of 6-mercaptopurine on antibody production. *Proc. Soc. Exp. Biol. Med.*, 99:164–167.

Schwartz, W. B. (1949), The effect of sulfanilamide on salt and water excretion in congestive heart failure. *New Engl. J. Med.*, 240:173–177.

Schwidetzky, O. (1944), History of needles and syringes. *Curr. Res. Anesth. Analg.*, 23:34–38.

Scott, D. A., & Charles, A. F. (1933), Studies on heparin III. The purification of heparin. *J. Biol. Chem.*, 102:437–448.

Scott, E. L. (1911–1912), On the influence of intravenous injections of an extract of the pancreas on experimental pancreatic diabetes. *Amer. J. Physiol.*, 29:306–310.

Seguin, E. (1866–1867), Clinical thermometry. *Med. Record*, 1:516–519.

——— (1876), *Medical Thermometry and Human Temperature*. New York: William Wood & Co.

Sen, G., & Bose, K. C. (1931), Rawolfia serpentina: A new Indian drug for insanity and high blood pressure. *Indian Med. World*, 2:194–201.

Sertürner, F. W. A. (1817), On morphium, a salt-like base, and meconic acid as chief constituents of opium. In: *Drug Discovery: The Evolution of Modern Medicines*, by W. Sneader. Chichester, New York, Brisbane, Toronto, Singapore: John Wiley & Sons, 1985, p. 7.

Shakespeare, W. (n.d.), *The Complete Works of William Shakespeare*, ed. W. J. Craig. London: Oxford University Press, 1943.

Shanks, R. G. (1984), The discovery of beta-adrenoceptor blocking drugs. *Trends Pharmacol. Sci.*, 5:405–409.

Shattock, S. G. (1900), Chromocyte clumping in acute pneumonia and certain other diseases, and the significance of the buffy coat in the shed blood. *J. Pathol. Bacteriol.*, 6:303–314.

Shoemaker, J. V. (1901), The therapeutic benefit of music. *Med. Bull.*, 23:290–294.

Siegel, R. E., & Poynter, F. N. L. (1962), Robert Talbor, Charles II, and cinchona: A contemporary document. *Med. Hist.*, 6:82–85.

Sigerist, H. E. (1933), *The Great Doctors: A Biographical History of Medicine*, trans. E. & C. Paul. New York: Dover Publications, Inc., 1971.

——— (1943), *Civilization and Disease*. Chicago & London: University of Chicago Press, 1962.

Smith, E. (1857), The influence of the labour of the treadwheel over respiration and pulsation. *Med. Times & Gazette*, N. S. 14:601–603.

Smith, E. L., & Parker, L. F. J. (1948), Purification of anti-pernicious anaemia factor. In: Proceedings of the Biochemical Society, 1948. *Biochem. J.*, 43:viii–ix.

Smith, F. M. (1918), The ligation of coronary arteries with electrocardiographic study. *Arch. Intern. Med.*, 22:8–27.

Smith, J. L. (1899), The pathological effects due to increase of oxygen tension in the air breathed. *J. Physiol.*, 24:19–35.

Sneader, W. (1985), *Drug Discovery: The Evolution of Modern Medicines*. Chichester, New York, Brisbane, Toronto, Singapore: John Wiley & Sons.

Solandt, D. Y., & Best, C. H. (1938), Heparin and coronary thrombosis in experimental animals. *Lancet*, 2:130–132.

Souttar, H. S. (1925), The surgical treatment of mitral stenosis. *Brit. Med. J.*, 2:603–606.

Stadie, W. C. (1919), The oxygen of the arterial and venous blood in pneumonia and its relation to cyanosis. *J. Exp. Med.*, 30:215–240.

——— (1922), Construction of an oxygen chamber for the treatment of pneumonia. *J. Exp. Med.*, 35:323–335.

——— Riggs, B. C., & Haugaard, N. (1944), Oxygen poisoning. *Amer. J. Med. Sci.*, 207:84–114.

Stahmann, M. A., Huebner, C. F., & Link, K. P. (1941), Studies on the hemorrhagic sweet clover disease. V. Identification and synthesis of the hemorrhagic agent. *J. Biol. Chem.*, 138:513–527.

Stanley, E. (1873), The Conduct of Life, address at Liverpool College. In: *Familiar Medical Quotations*, ed. M. B. Strauss. Boston: Little, Brown & Co., 1968, p. 165.

Stannard, J. (1974), Squill in ancient and medieval materia medica, with special reference to its employment for dropsy. *Bull. New York Acad. Med.*, 50:684–713.

Starr, A., & Edwards, M. L. (1961), Mitral replacement: Clinical experience with a ball-valve prosthesis. *Ann. Surg.*, 154:726–740.

Steell, G. (1888), The murmur of high-pressure in the pulmonary artery. *Med. Chronicle, Manchester*, 9:182–188.

Stephenson, Jr., H. E. (1974), *Cardiac Arrest and Resuscitation*. St. Louis: C. V. Mosby Co.

Stockman, R. (1893), The treatment of chlorosis by iron and some other drugs. *Brit. Med. J.*, 1:881–885.

Stokes, W. (1825), *An Introduction to the Use of the Stethoscope*. Edinburgh: Maclachlan & Stewart.

────── (1854), *The Diseases of the Heart and the Aorta*. Dublin: Hodges & Smith.

Swan, H., & Schechter, D. C. (1962), The transfusion of blood from cadavers: A historical review. *Surgery*, 52:545–560.

Sydenham, T. (1676), Medical observations concerning the history and the cure of acute diseases. In: *The Works of Thomas Sydenham, M.D.*, Vol. 1, ed. R. G. Latham. London: The Sydenham Society, 1848, pp. 1–276.

────── (1682), Epistolary dissertation to Dr. Cole. In: *The Works of Thomas Sydenham, M.D.*, Vol. 2, ed. R. G. Latham. London: The Sydenham Society, 1850, pp. 51–118.

────── (1683), A treatise on gout, and dropsy. In: *The Works of Thomas Sydenham, M.D.*, Vol. 2, ed. R. G. Latham. London: The Sydenham Society, 1850, pp. 119–184.

Tannahill, R. (1973), *Food in History*. New York: Stein and Day.

Taussig, H. B. (1947), *Congenital Malformations of the Heart*. New York: The Commonwealth Fund.

Taylor, F. S. (1942), The origin of the thermometer. *Ann. Sci.*, 5:129–156.

Tennyson, A. (1847), The Princess; a Medley. In: *The Complete Poetical Works of Tennyson*, ed. W. J. Rolfe. Boston: Houghton Mifflin Company, 1898, pp. 115–162.

The Holy Bible: Revised Standard Version Containing the Old and New Testaments, ed. H. G. May & B. M. Metzger. New York: Oxford University Press, 1962.

The Medical News (1887), Editorial: Calomel as a diuretic. *The Medical News*, 50:268.

────── (1888), Editorial: Calomel as a diuretic. *The Medical News*, 53:593.

Tissot, J.-C. (1780), *Gymnastique Médicinale et Chirurgicale*, trans. E. & S. Licht. New Haven, CT: Elizabeth Licht, Publisher, 1964.

Tovell, R. M., & Remlinger, Jr., J. E. (1941), History and present status of oxygen therapy and resuscitation. *J. Amer. Med. Assn.*, 117:1939–1943.

Turner, T. B., Bennett, V. L., & Hernandez, H. (1981), The beneficial side of moderate alcohol use. *The Johns Hopkins Med. J.*, 148:53–63.

Tyler, V. E., Brady, L. R., & Robbers, J. E. (1981), *Pharmacognosy*. Philadelphia: Lea & Febiger.

Vakil, R. J. (1949), A clinical trial of Rauwolfia serpentina in essential hypertension. *Brit. Heart J.*, 11:350–355.

Van Slyke, D. D. (1918), Gasometric determination of the oxygen and hemoglobin of blood. *J. Biol. Chem.*, 33:127–132.

Veith, I. (1949), *Huang Ti Nei Ching Su Wên—The Yellow Emperor's Classic of Internal Medicine*. Berkeley & Los Angeles: University of California Press, 1966.

Velebit, V., Podrid, P., Lown, B., Cohen, B. H., & Graboys, T. B. (1982), Aggravation and provocation of ventricular arrhythmias by antiarrhythmic drugs. *Circulation*, 65:886–894.

Vincent, S., & Thompson, J. H. (1929), The effects of music upon the human blood pressure. *Lancet*, 1:534–537.

Vineberg, A. M. (1946), Development of an anastomosis between the coronary vessels and a transplanted internal mammary artery. *Can. Med. Assn. J.*, 55:117–119.

Vogl, A. (1950), The discovery of the organic mercurial diuretics. *Amer. Heart J.*, 39:881–883.

Von Mering, J., & Minkowski, O. (1889), Diabetes mellitus after extirpation of the pancreas. In: *Classic Descriptions of Disease*, ed. R. H. Major. Springfield, IL, & Baltimore, MD: Charles C Thomas, 1932, pp. 204–208.

Von Niemeyer, F. (1881), A *Textbook of Practical Medicine*, Vol. 2, trans. G. H. Humphreys & C. E. Hackley. New York: D. Appleton & Company.

Von Stoerck, A. (1764), *An Essay on the Use and Effect of the Root of the Colchicum Autumnale, or Meadow-Saffron*. London: T. Becket & P. A. DeHondt.

Wallace, S. L. (1968), Benjamin Franklin and the introduction of colchicum into the United States. *Bull. Hist. Med.*, 42:312–320.

Waller, A. D. (1887), A demonstration on man of electromotive changes accompanying the heart's beat. *J. Physiol.*, 8:229–234.

Want, J. (1815), Composition of Eau médicinale (abstract). *New Engl. J. Med. Surg.*, 4:88–90.

Wardner, L. H. (1988), The world's longest insulin patient. *Cornell Univ. Med. College Alumni Q.*, 49 (No. 4):30–34.

Webster, Jr., L. T. (1985), Drugs used in the chemotherapy of protozoal infections. In: *Goodman and Gilman's the Pharmacologic Basis of Therapeutics*, ed. A. G. Gilman, L. S. Goodman, T. W. Rall, & F. Murad. New York: Macmillan Publishing Co., pp. 1029–1048.

Weiner, N. (1985), Drugs that inhibit adrenergic nerves and block adrenergic receptors. In: *Goodman and Gilman's the Pharmacologic Basis of Therapeutics*, ed. A. G. Gilman, L. S. Goodman, T. W. Rall, & F. Murad. New York: Macmillan Publishing Co., pp. 181–214.

Weirich, W. L., Gott, V. L., & Lillehei, C. W. (1957), The treatment of complete heart block by the combined use of a myocardial electrode and an artificial pacemaker. *Surg. Forum*, 8:360–363.

Wells, P. N. T. (1978), History. In: *Handbook of Clinical Ultrasound*, ed. M. de Vlieger, J. H. Holmes, E. Kazner, G. Kossoff, A. Kratochwil, R. Kraus, J. Poujol, & D. E. Strandness. New York, Chichester, Brisbane, Toronto: John Wiley & Sons, pp. 3–13.

Wenckebach, K. F. (1923), Cinchona derivatives in the treatment of heart disorders. *J. Amer. Med. Assn.*, 81:472–474.

West, R. (1948), Activity of vitamin B_{12} in Addisonian pernicious anemia. *Science*, 107:398.

Whipple, G. H., Robscheit, F. S., & Hooper, C. W. (1920), Blood regeneration
    following simple anemia IV. Influence of meat, liver, and various extractives,
    alone or combined with standard diets. *Amer. J. Physiol.*, 53:236–262.
White, D. N. (1982), Johann Christian Doppler and his effect—A brief history.
    Ultrasound Med. Biol., 8:583–591.
White, P. D. (1944), *Heart Disease.* New York: The Macmillan Company.
—— (1972), Place of exercise in cardiology. *Amer. J. Cardiol.*, 30:716–717.
—— Marvin, H. M., & Burwell, C. S. (1921), The action of quinidine sulphate
    in heart disease, to abolish the circus movement of auricular flutter and fi-
    brillation. *Boston Med. Surg. J.*, 185:647–650.
Wiggers, C. J., & Wégria, R. (1940), Ventricular fibrillation due to single, localized
    induction and condenser shocks applied during the vulnerable phase of ven-
    tricular systole. *Amer. J. Physiol.*, 128:500–505.
Wild, J. J., & Reid, J. M. (1952), Further pilot echographic studies on the histologic
    structure of tumors of the living intact human breast. *Amer. J. Path.*,
    28:839–861.
—— —— (1956), Diagnostic use of ultrasound. *Brit. J. Physical Med.*,
    19:248–257, 264.
Wilkes, E., & Levy, J., eds. (1984), *Advances in Morphine Therapy: The 1983
    International Symposium on Pain Control* (International Congress and Sym-
    posium Series; No. 64). London: The Royal Society of Medicine.
Wilkins, R. W. (1953), Hypertension: Recent trends in treatment. *Med. Clin. North
    Amer.*, 37:1303–1312.
—— (1954), Current therapeutics LXXIX.—Rauwolfia serpentina. *The Practi-
    tioner*, 173:84–89.
Wilks, S. (1903), The early history of clinical thermometry. *Brit. Med. J.*,
    1:1058–1059.
Willis, T. (1679), Pharmaceutice Rationalis or an Exercitation of the Operations of
    Medicines in Humane Bodies. In: *Classic Descriptions of Disease*, ed. R. H.
    Major. Springfield, IL, & Baltimore, MD: Charles C Thomas, 1932, pp.
    192–194.
Willius, F. A., & Keys, T. E. (1941), *Cardiac Classics.* St. Louis: C. V. Mosby Co.
—— —— (1942), Cardiac clinics XCIV. A remarkably early reference to the
    use of cinchona in cardiac arrhythmia. *Proc. Staff Meetings Mayo Clin.*,
    17:294–296.
Willman, V. L., Cooper, T., Cian, L. G., & Hanlon, C. R. (1962), Autotrans-
    plantation of the canine heart. *Surg. Gynec., Obst.*, 115:299–302.
Wilson, F. N., & Herrmann, G. R. (1920), Bundle branch block and arborization
    block. *Arch. Intern. Med.*, 26:153–191.
Wimmer, S. J. (1889), The influence of music and its therapeutic value. *New York
    Med. J.*, 50:258–260.
Withering, W. (1785), *An Account of the Foxglove, and Some of its Medical Uses:
    With Practical Remarks on Dropsy, and Other Diseases.* London: G. G. J.
    & J. Robinson.
Wolff, L., Parkinson, J., & White, P. D. (1930), Bundle-branch block with short
    P-R interval in healthy young people prone to paroxysmal tachycardia. *Amer.
    Heart J.*, 5:685–704.
Wood, A. (1855), New method of treating neuralgia by the direct application of
    opiates to the painful points. *Edinburgh Med. Surg. J.*, 82:265–281.

——— (1858), Treatment of neuralgic pains by narcotic injections. *Brit. Med. J.*, 1858:721–723.

Wood, P. (1956), *Diseases of the Heart and Circulation*. London: Eyre & Spottiswoode.

Woods, R. H. (1906), On artificial respiration. *Trans. R. Acad. Med. Ireland*, 24:136–141.

Woodson, Jr., R. E., Youngken, H. W., Schlittler, E., & Schneider, J. A. (1957), *Rauwolfia: Botany, Pharmacognosy, Chemistry & Pharmacology*. Boston, Toronto: Little, Brown and Company.

Wordsworth, W. (1807), Resolution and Independence. In: The *Poetical Works of William Wordsworth*, ed. T. Hutchinson. London: Oxford University Press, 1920, pp. 195–197.

Wright, A. D. (1968), The history of opium. *Med. Biol. Ill.*, 18:62–70.

Wright, I. S., & Prandoni, A. (1942), The dicoumarin 3,3'-methylene-bis(4-hydroxycoumarin): Its pharmacologic and therapeutic action in man. *J. Amer. Med. Assn.*, 120:1015–1021.

Wunderlich, C. A. (1868), *On the Temperature in Diseases: A Manual of Medical Thermometry*, trans. W. B. Woodman. London: New Sydenham Society, 1871.

Yudin, S. S. (1936), Transfusion of cadaver blood. *J. Amer. Med. Assn.*, 106:997–999.

Zipes, D. P. (1985), A consideration of antiarrhythmic therapy. *Circulation*, 72:949–956.

Zoll, P. M. (1952), Resuscitation of the heart in ventricular standstill by external electric stimulation. *New Engl. J. Med.*, 247:768–771.

——— Frank, H. A., Zarsky, L. R. N., Linenthal, A. J., & Belgard, A. H. (1961), Long-term electric stimulation of the heart for Stokes-Adams disease. *Ann. Surg.*, 154:330–346.

——— Linenthal, A. J., Gibson, W., Paul, M. H., & Norman, L. R. (1956), Termination of ventricular fibrillation in man by externally applied electric countershock. *New Engl. J. Med.*, 254:727–732.

——— ——— Norman, L. R. (1954), Treatment of Stokes-Adams disease by external electric stimulation of the heart. *Circulation*, 9:482–493.

Name Index

Abbott, M. E., 184
Abel, J. J., 108, 121
Acosta, C., 86
Addison, J., 141
Addison, T., 93, 97
Aesculapius (legendary Greek physician), 125; *see* Asclepius
Ahlquist, R. P., 174, 175, 177
Aldini, J., 187
Aldobrandino da Siena, 134
Alexander of Tralles, 81
Allbutt, T. C., 46
Allen, E. V., 152
Altshuler, I. M., 130
Antyllos (Greco-Roman surgeon), 118
Apollo (Greek god), 125
Arena, J. M., 87
Aretaeus the Cappadocian, 103
Aristotle, 2, 55
Arnald of Villanova, 134
Arthus, M., 23
Asclepiades (ancient Greek physician), 126
Asclepius, 125, 130; *see* Aesculapius
Atropos (Greek mythology), 88
Auenbrugger, L., 32, 35
Auer, J., 180
Aurelianus, C., 126, 142
Avicenna, 68, 74, 118, 133

Baer, J. E., 96
Baglivi, G., 127
Bailey, C. P., 185
Baker, A. B., 3-4, 5
Baker, C., 185

Banting, F. G., 105-106, 107
Barach, A. L., 114
Barcroft, J., 111, 113
Barker, F., 30
Barnard, C. N., 205
Barnard, H., 52, 53*f*
Bartholow, R., 86, 89, 92, 94, 135, 168, 169
Battelli, F., 12
Beaumont, W., 188
Beck, C. S., 13, 183-184
Beddoes, T., 110-111
Benedek, T. G., 79, 80, 81, 82
Bernard, C., 50, 182
Bernstein, J., 56
Berridge, V., 69
Bert, P., 115
Best, C. H., 106, 107, 150
Beverley, R., 86-87
Beyer, K. H., Jr., 96
Biddle, J. B., 74, 86, 92, 94, 135
Biermer, A., 98
Bigelow, W. G., 185, 191, 193
Billroth, T., 179
Bingham, J. B., 152
Birtwell, W. C., 197
Black, J. W., 175, 176, 177
Black, M. M., 200
Blaiberg, P., 205
Blalock, A., 184-185
Blaud, P., 75-76
Bleichroeder, F., 182
Bliss, M., 106, 107, 108
Bloebaum, F., 89
Blumgart, H. L., 95

239

Subject Index

Amyl nitrite, 162-163, 165-166
  for angina pectoris, 162-163, 166
  compared with nitroglycerine, 165-166
  studies on, 162-163
Anemia; *see* Chlorosis; Iron therapy; Pernicious anemia
Angina pectoris, 62, 70, 161-166, 175, 176
  description of, 161-162; *see also Commentaries on the History and Cure of Diseases*
  surgery for, 183-184
  treatment of with wine, 134-135
  see also Amyl nitrite; Beta-adrenergic blocking agents; Nitroglycerine
Anticoagulants, 149-153; *see also* Dicumarol; Heparin; Hirudin; Warfarin
Arterial puncture in humans
  for blood gas analysis, 112-113
  for recording blood pressure, 50
Artificial respiration, 3-6
  in antiquity, 3-6
  manual methods of, 5-6
  mouth-to-airway methods of, 4-5, 6, 9
  Vesalius and, 3-4
Atropa belladona (deadly nightshade), 83, 88
  derivation of the name, 88
  in a sixteenth century herbal, 88
Auscultation
  direct (immediate), 31, 32-33, 38
  indirect (mediate); *see* Stethoscope
Austin Flint murmur; 38; *see also* Stethoscope

Babylonian Talmud, 132; *see also* Wine, medical uses of
Belladona alkaloids, 83-90
  clinical uses and effects of, 88-90
  and the nightshade family of plants; *see also Atropa belladona; Datura stramonium; Hyoscyamus niger; Mandragora officinarum*
Beta-adrenergic blocking agents (beta blockers), 173-177
  for cardiac disorders, 175-177
  experimental origins of, 173-175
  selective blockade with, 176-177
  see also Pronethalol (nethalide); Propranolol
Blood, ingestion of
  for nutrition, 15
  for strength and health, 15
Blood pressure, measurement of, 49-54
  by auscultatory method of Korotkov, 52, 54
  direct arterial, 49-50
  early instrument for, 53*f*
  experimental, 49-50
  noninvasive (indirect), 50-54
Blood transfusions, 15-24
  animal-to-animal, 16-17
  animal-to-man, 17, 18*f*, 19
  blood banks and, 23-24
  Blundell's procedure for human, 19, 20, 21*f*
  cadaver blood for, 24
  methods to prevent clotting of, 23-24
  reactions to, 19-20, 22
  as recorded in Pepys' diary, 17
  typing and cross-matching of, 22

247